REPORT

T0302545

The Abuse of Medical Diagnostic Practices in Mass Litigation

The Case of Silica

Stephen J. Carroll, Lloyd Dixon, James M. Anderson, Thor Hogan, Elizabeth M. Sloss

RAND INSTITUTE FOR CIVIL JUSTICE

The research described in this report was conducted by the RAND Institute of Civil Justice, a unit of the RAND Corporation. This research was supported by the National Industrial Sand Association, the U.S. Chamber of Commerce Institute for Legal Reform, and the Coalition for Litigation Justice.

Library of Congress Cataloging-in-Publication Data

The abuse of medical diagnostic practices in mass litigation : the case of silica / Stephen J. Carroll, Lloyd Dixon, James M. Anderson, Thor Hogan, Elizabeth M. Sloss.
p. cm.
"This research was supported by the RAND Institute for Civil Justice, the National Industrial Sand Association, the U.S. Chamber of Commerce Institute for Legal Reform, and the Coalition for Litigation Justice."
Includes bibliographical references.
ISBN 978-0-8330-4912-4 (pbk. : alk. paper)
1. Industrial safety—Law and legislation—United States. 2. Silicosis—Law and legislation—United States. 3. Class actions (Civil procedure)—United States—Corrupt practices. 4. Evidence, Expert—United States—Corrupt practices. 5. Medical jurisprudence—United States—Corrupt practices. I. Carroll, Stephen J., 1940– II. Institute for Civil Justice (U.S.)

KF3570.A72 2009
344.7304'65—dc22

2009045739

The RAND Corporation is a nonprofit research organization providing objective analysis and effective solutions that address the challenges facing the public and private sectors around the world. RAND's publications do not necessarily reflect the opinions of its research clients and sponsors.

RAND® is a registered trademark.

Published 2009 by the RAND Corporation
1776 Main Street, P.O. Box 2138, Santa Monica, CA 90407-2138
1200 South Hayes Street, Arlington, VA 22202-5050
4570 Fifth Avenue, Suite 600, Pittsburgh, PA 15213-2665
RAND URL: http://www.rand.org/
To order RAND documents or to obtain additional information, contact
Distribution Services: Telephone: (310) 451-7002;
Fax: (310) 451-6915; Email: order@rand.org

Preface

Litigation over injuries due to the inhalation of respirable silica dust in the workplace skyrocketed beginning in 2001, raising concerns that silica litigation would become a mass tort with similarities to the asbestos litigation that had occurred in the previous 30 years. However, the silica litigation collapsed soon after the discovery of numerous abuses in the procedures used to diagnose the injuries.

The uncovering of grossly inadequate diagnostic practices was a significant success for the tort system in handling a mass tort. However, there is no guarantee that similar practices would be uncovered should they be used in the future. This report reviews the court proceedings that led to the uncovering of abusive diagnostic practices in silica litigation. The insights are then used to identify several areas in which changes in litigation practices and procedures could increase the likelihood that similar diagnostic practices would be uncovered in the future or prevented from occurring in the first place.

This report should be of interest to federal and state policymakers, lawyers, judges, and litigants concerned about the reliability of medical diagnoses and other expert evidence in mass personal-injury litigation. The changes suggested in this study might be used as a starting point for discussions among stakeholders on how to improve the tort system.

This research was supported by the RAND Institute for Civil Justice, the National Industrial Sand Association, the U.S. Chamber of Commerce Institute for Legal Reform, and the Coalition for Litigation Justice. The views in the report are those of the authors and do not necessarily reflect those of the research sponsors.

The RAND Institute for Civil Justice

The mission of the RAND Institute for Civil Justice (ICJ) is to improve private and public decisionmaking on civil legal issues by supplying policymakers and the public with the results of objective, empirically based, analytic research. ICJ facilitates change in the civil justice system by analyzing trends and outcomes, identifying and evaluating policy options, and bringing together representatives of different interests to debate alternative solutions to policy problems. ICJ builds on a long tradition of RAND research characterized by an interdisciplinary, empirical approach to public policy issues and rigorous standards of quality, objectivity, and independence.

ICJ research is supported by pooled grants from corporations, trade and professional associations, and individuals; by government grants and contracts; and by private foundations. ICJ disseminates its work widely to the legal, business, and research communities and to the general public. In accordance with RAND policy, all ICJ research products are subject to peer review before publication. ICJ publications do not necessarily reflect the opinions or policies of the research sponsors or of the ICJ Board of Overseers.

Information about ICJ is available online (http://www.rand.org/icj/). Inquiries about research projects should be sent to the following address:

James Dertouzos, Director
RAND Institute for Civil Justice
1776 Main Street
P.O. Box 2138
Santa Monica, CA 90407-2138
310-393–0411 x7476
Fax: 310-451-6979
James_Dertouzos@rand.org

Questions and comments about this report should be sent to Lloyd Dixon (Lloyd_Dixon@rand.org).

Contents

Figures

Summary

From 2001 to 2003, claims for injuries caused by inhaling silica dust skyrocketed, and commentators began to describe silica in terms of asbestos: It had the potential to be a mass tort that would last for decades. Within two years, however, the litigation was essentially over. In 2003, more than 10,000 claims—about 100 cases against 250 defendants—were aggregated in the Southern District of Texas before U.S. District Court Judge Janis Graham Jack to determine whether the federal courts had jurisdiction based on diversity. The proceeding in Judge Jack's court exposed gross abuses in the diagnosing of silica-related injuries, and, due in large part to her findings, the litigation collapsed.

In this report, we analyze the proceedings in Judge Jack's courtroom to identify how the widespread abuse was discovered. Besides describing the actions and decisions of the judge herself, we take a broad look at the behavior of attorneys and the characteristics of the litigation that contributed to the outcome. In the end, we consider what can be learned from the silica experience that might improve the ability of the civil justice system to detect the abuse of medical diagnostic practices in mass personal-injury litigation. Although we have not done the analysis needed to support specific policy recommendations, we identify the types of changes that should be analyzed by researchers and considered by policymakers to strengthen the performance of the tort system in this regard.

We base our analysis on data and knowledge gained in previous RAND research on asbestos and other mass toxic tort litigation, a detailed review of the proceedings before Judge Jack, data on silica-related claims from a major defendant in the silica litigation, and interviews with 43 individuals who have been involved in various aspects of silica litigation or mass torts more generally.

The Exposure of Diagnostic Abuses in Silica Litigation

A sequence of events occurred in Judge Jack's court that led to the exposure of gross deficiencies in the diagnoses underlying the silica claims in front of her. In January 2004, Judge Jack issued a discovery order that required each plaintiff to submit a sworn fact sheet specifying the plaintiff's diagnosis and pertinent medical and diagnostic information, as well as the results of B-reads of chest x-rays.[1] The fact sheets revealed that more than 9,000 plaintiffs were diagnosed by only 12 doctors and that a substantial fraction of the plaintiffs in the silica multidistrict litigation (MDL) had earlier filed claims for asbestos-related injuries.

Plaintiffs opposed defense requests to depose the diagnosing doctors and the three medical screening firms associated with the cases. Before Judge Jack could rule on motions to quash the discovery requests, one of the doctors agreed to be deposed and testified that he had never diagnosed silicosis. Judge Jack then ordered every doctor who diagnosed silicosis in any of the plaintiffs and two of the three medical screening companies to testify at a *Daubert* hearing in front of the court.[2]

At the hearing, Judge Jack questioned representatives from each of two medical screening companies and several diagnosing doctors. She concluded that virtually all of the diagnoses failed to satisfy the minimum, medically acceptable criteria for the diagnosis of silicosis. Exposure and health histories had been taken by people who not only had no medical training but had a financial interest in the outcome of a diagnosis. The diagnosing doctors relied solely on x-rays and failed to rule out other explanations for x-ray evidence or lung distress.

Judge Jack remanded all but one case to state court, citing lack of jurisdiction. However, the order doing so questioned the validity of virtually every claim. The court criticized the procedures used by the doctors who had diagnosed the vast majority of the plaintiffs and ordered sanctions against the plaintiffs' firm for the case for which she retained jurisdiction, finding that its behavior had been unreasonable and vexatious.[3]

Silica litigation plummeted following Judge Jack's order. Plaintiffs' firms voluntarily dismissed the bulk of the silica claims remanded to Texas and Mississippi state courts. Legal reforms enacted in several states during this period likely contributed to the decline in claims, but Jack's findings were undoubtedly a driving factor in the end of silica as a mass tort.

The impact of the ruling also spread to asbestos litigation. For example, the Manville Trust, one of the major trusts set up by the courts to pay asbestos claims, saw a major decline in claims and announced that it would no longer accept medical reports in support of asbestos claims from most of the doctors and testing facilities behind the diagnoses in the cases considered by Judge Jack. One of the doctors suspended by

---

[1] B-reads are done by physicians that have been certified through the B-reader program of the National Institute for Occupational Safety and Health (NIOSH). The program certifies that doctors are trained to interpret pulmonary x-rays using the International Labour Organization (ILO) International Classification of Radiographs of Pneumoconiosis.

[2] *Daubert v. Merrell Dow Pharms.* (509 U.S. 579, 1993) was a U.S. Supreme Court decision that became the basis for a judge's review of the admissibility of expert testimony—a *Daubert* hearing.

[3] She may have had similar views on the behavior of the other plaintiffs' firms involved in the litigation but was silent, given that she remanded the other cases to state court.

Manville, Ray Harron, had submitted documents in support of at least 53,724 of the approximately 680,000 claims that the Manville Trust had received through 2005.

Factors That Contributed to Exposure of Diagnostic Abuses in Silica Litigation

To understand how the tort system succeeded in exposing the grossly inadequate diagnostic practices in the silica setting, we identify factors that worked in favor of as well as factors that worked against exposing the diagnostic abuses. In the case of silica, the factors that worked in favor of uncovering such practices won out, but such may not be the case in other settings.

Actions by the Defense

Three defense strategies were particularly important in the discovery of abuses in silica diagnoses. First, defendants succeeded in removing cases filed in Mississippi and Texas state courts to federal court, where they could be brought together in front of one judge. Because of this aggregation, defendants were able to see that a small number of doctors accounted for a huge number of the diagnoses. Second, the defense attorneys challenged the diagnoses, something that does not always happen. And third, the leading defense firm built detailed databases on a large number of silica and asbestos claims, including claims that were not part of the litigation before Judge Jack. The data showed that a vast number of plaintiffs had previously filed asbestos claims.

These strategies were hotly contested among the defense attorneys. According to defense counsel involved with the case, some attorneys were opposed to the confrontational tactics of Forman Perry Watkins Krutz and Tardy, the lead defense firm. Some opposed aggregation by arguing that removing so many cases to a single court would risk an assignment to a plaintiff-friendly federal district court or that discovery in federal district court could aid plaintiffs' attorneys in bringing other cases. Some attorneys proposed settling claims rather than challenging the diagnoses, on the grounds that challenging them could add to legal costs or even to reprisals by plaintiffs' attorneys. The third strategy, building the database, was an expensive undertaking that was made possible by two factors: advances in computer software and the fact that the lead defense firm represented a large number of defendants that could spread the costs.

Procedural Decisions by Judge Jack

Several of Judge Jack's decisions stand in sharp contrast to the judicial procedures often used in such cases. First, requiring fact sheets with every plaintiff's diagnosis and all pertinent medical and diagnostic information early in the case provided defense attorneys with information that was essential to uncovering diagnostic irregularities. More commonly, plaintiffs' attorneys do not provide a physician's diagnosis until discovery, and, if the case settles, a diagnosis may never be provided.

Second, Judge Jack not only allowed the diagnosing doctors to be deposed by defense attorneys, she directed the depositions to occur in her presence in the form of a *Daubert* hearing. Leading defense attorneys interviewed for this study commented that the latitude to question doctors across all the plaintiffs in front of a judge was unprecedented. The presence of the judge reduced the number of plaintiff objections and resulted in more-direct answers. Judge Jack also actively participated in the cross-examination and heard firsthand about the diagnostic practices underlying the claims.

Third, Judge Jack actively managed the case. She called for early disclosure of diagnoses, required the doctors to testify in her presence (to address allegations made by both sides of misconduct during depositions), and held a monthly status conference with opposing counsel. This active case management contrasts with judicial case management in other settings described by those interviewed: When faced with a large number of claims and a crowded docket, judges often allow cases to churn for a few years in hopes that they will settle.

Unique Characteristics of Silica Litigation

Some features of the litigation itself contributed to the discovery of diagnostic abuses:

- a large number of cases and the preexistence of litigation in a closely related area (asbestos)
- the absence of a terminal cancer uniquely associated with silica, which reduced defendant concerns about cases coming to trial and about plaintiffs' attorneys' threats to target defendants who challenged diagnoses.

Policy Implications

The federal court's actions and the consequences of those actions clearly demonstrate that the tort system has the capacity to identify questionable claims in a mass-tort setting. However, one should not be too satisfied with the performance of the tort system in this regard. First, the diagnostic practices were attempted in the first place, and considerable time and expense were spent in exposing them. Second, the tort system does not appear to have been nearly so effective in the largest mass tort to date—asbestos litigation. For example, it is reasonable to suspect that many of the asbestos claims based on Harron's reports relied on similar procedures used in silica litigation.

There is thus no guarantee that similar practices would be discovered should they be used in the future. A number of factors worked in favor of uncovering diagnostic abuses in the silica litigation, and, absent the fortuitous alignment of these factors, litigation based on abusive diagnostic practices might have continued.

Our review of silica litigation generates some insights as to the types of changes in legal procedure and practice that have the potential to increase the likelihood that abusive diagnostic practices will be uncovered in future mass personal-injury litigation and improve the quality of the medical diagnoses that are introduced in the first place. If policymakers and practitioners agree that further improvements to the legal system in this area are needed, the pros and cons of the proposed changes should be carefully evaluated. Because the suggestions are based primarily on review of one type of litigation, an examination of experiences in other types of litigation would provide increased confidence about whether the benefits of change would outweigh their monetary and other costs. In addition, many of the changes we suggest for consideration raise important legal issues that should be more thoroughly explored: There may be need for modifications in the law and the rules of civil procedure at both the federal and state levels, and any changes might raise a variety of complex issues. Finally, it is important that the impact of potential changes on the ability of truly injured parties to pursue remedies in the civil justice system be considered.

We first discuss changes that focus on court procedures and practices. We then turn to changes aimed at influencing the behavior of plaintiff and defense lawyers.

Judicial Practices and Procedures

Require Diagnosis to Be Provided with Relevant Medical Records at Time of Case Filing. Requiring disclosure of the diagnosis, the identity of the diagnosing physician, and relevant medical records at case filing as soon as the litigation has achieved a sufficient size would help ensure adherence to defensible diagnostic practices and allow defendants to more rapidly evaluate and value claims.

Require Parties Early On to Present Evidence on Appropriate Diagnostic Practices and Whether They Were Followed. Once litigation has reached a sufficient scale, courts should require evidence that diagnoses were based on reasonable medical standards or consistent with accepted medical practice. Such a determination could be accomplished with briefs submitted by defense and plaintiffs' lawyers or by hearings in front of the court. If a substantial number of claims are based on diagnosis from a particular doctor, the court could consider conducting a hearing on the doctor's training, any affiliation with the screening facilities involved with the claims, and the procedures followed in his or her practice.

Augment Guidance for Multidistrict Litigation Judges. There are strong differences of opinion in the legal community about the proactive role that Judge Jack played in this case. For that reason, we suggest that more guidance be provided for federal and state judges on how they should handle mass personal-injury torts. For example, it may be appropriate to expand the Federal Judicial Center's (2004) *Manual for Complex Litigation, Fourth*, to provide an assessment of what types of judicial practices have been effective in mass personal-injury litigation and which have not. The manual might identify a set of recommended practices for mass personal-injury cases.

Enhance Mechanisms for Aggregating Information Across Claims for Pretrial Purposes. Procedures exist for aggregating claims for pretrial purposes, such as discovery and evaluation of the evidence, but they have important limitations. The pros and cons of changes that would facilitate the aggregation of claims in mass personal-injury litigation for pretrial purposes should be explored. Options that warrant further consideration include the following:

- Create an infrastructure for voluntary coordination between state and federal judges.
- Create a mechanism that would allow federal courts to aggregate claims in state courts for the purpose of developing information about the cases.
- Facilitate consolidation of cases already in federal court.

Practices of the Plaintiffs' and Defense Bars

Consider More-Serious Sanctions for Pursuing Cases Based on Grossly Inadequate Diagnoses. Judge Jack fined one plaintiffs' firm the prorated share of the excess costs, expenses, and attorneys' fees that the defendants incurred for the *Daubert* hearing. However, the fine was so small that the direct financial consequences for the firm were minor, and subsequent defense motions in Mississippi state courts for sanctions against other plaintiffs' firms failed.

Judge Jack imposed sanctions under a section of the U.S. Code (28 U.S.C. §1927) that allows sanctions only for direct excess costs, but Rule 11 of the Federal Rules of Civil Procedure (F.R.C.P. 11) allows penalties that would deter improper behavior. Judges should routinely consider fines that would deter the behavior rather than just recover excess costs.

Policymakers might also consider strengthening Rule 11. Since 1993, penalties for improper attorney conduct are discretionary, and a return to the mandatory penalties that existed before 1993 should be considered. The tools available to state court judges for deterring improper attorney behavior should also be reviewed and assessed.

Pay Closer Attention to the Performance of the Defense Bar. While plaintiffs' firms are typically the focus of complaints about diagnostic practices, our investigation of silica litigation identified a number of defense-attorney practices that enabled litigation based on inadequate diagnoses. For example, one plaintiffs' attorney interviewed for this study recalled multiple instances in which a defense attorney would call and suggest that his client be named in a silica case.

It is not obvious how to deter defense practices that enable litigation based on inadequate diagnostic practices, in part because such practices are difficult to observe. For example, it is difficult to determine the extent to which a defense attorney is simply churning a claim to generate fees with the ultimate goal of settling, without any concerted effort to challenge suspect diagnoses. However, given the importance of the issue, policymakers and practitioners should seriously consider what types of responses might be effective. For example, policymakers and practitioners might consider developing means to chronicle and evaluate defense tactics in mass personal-injury litigation, including defense tactics directed by defendants' insurers. The results could motivate greater attention to ethical issues in law schools and continuing-education courses as well as in investigations by professional review panels.

Acknowledgments

Many people made important contributions to this project. We would first like to thank those who spent time with us to share their experiences about silica litigation. The interviews were done on a confidential basis, so we cannot thank them by name, but this report would not have been possible without their participation.

Peer reviews were provided by John Mendeloff at RAND and Mark Peterson of Legal Analysis Systems. Helpful comments on drafts were provided by Mark Behrens of Shook Hardy and Bacon; Fred Krutz of Forman Perry Watkins Krutz and Tardy; Christian Lahnstein of Munich Re; David Setter of Socha, Perczak, Setter and Anderson; Paul Rheingold of Rheingold, Valet, Rheingold, Shkolnik and McCartney; and John Ulizio of U.S. Silica. We thank them for their time.

At RAND, we thank Jim Dertouzos, Fred Kipperman, and Robert Reville, both for providing the resources needed to complete the project and for helping move the project to completion. We particularly want to thank Susan Gates, the ICJ quality-assurance director, for her persistence in moving this project through the peer-review process. Thanks are also due to Laura Zakaras for helping improve the presentation of the findings and Lisa Bernard for skillful editing.

Abbreviations

ACGIH	American Conference of Governmental Industrial Hygienists
BLS	Bureau of Labor Statistics
COPD	chronic obstructive pulmonary disease
F.R.C.P.	Federal Rule of Civil Procedure
HIPAA	Health Insurance Portability and Accountability Act
IARC	International Agency for Research on Cancer
ILO	International Labour Organization
MDL	multidistrict litigation
NIOSH	National Institute for Occupational Safety and Health
NORMS	National Occupational Respiratory Mortality System
OSHA	Occupational Safety and Health Administration
PEL	permissible exposure limit
REL	recommended exposure limit
SENSOR	Sentinel Event Notification System for Occupational Risks
SIC	standard industrial classification
SiO_2	silicon dioxide
TB	tuberculosis
TLV	threshold limit value
TWA	time-weighted average

CHAPTER ONE

Introduction

In 2005, Judge Janis Jack, a federal judge in the Southern District of Texas, issued an order that effectively ended silica as a mass tort. Claims for injuries due to the inhalation of silica dust had remained at modest levels through the 1990s but then skyrocketed beginning in 2001, raising concerns that silica litigation would become a mass tort similar to the asbestos litigation that had occurred in the previous 30 years. The proceeding in Judge Jack's court uncovered gross abuses in the diagnosis of silica-related injuries, and her 2005 order focused national attention on problematic aspects of how silica claims entered and proceeded through the civil justice system. Due in large part to proceedings in Judge Jack's court, the litigation collapsed.

It may well be that policymakers and practitioners have learned enough from the silica experience that the United States will never again see mass litigation over injuries based on abusive diagnostic practices. But we cannot be sure. The prospect of large financial gain provides a powerful incentive to utilize inappropriate diagnostic procedures in order to manufacture large numbers of claims.

The uncovering of grossly inadequate diagnostic practices was a significant success for the tort system in handling a mass tort. The federal court's actions and the consequences of those actions clearly demonstrate that the tort system has the capacity to identify questionable claims in a mass tort setting. However, such an outcome is not guaranteed should similar practices be attempted in the future. A number of factors worked in favor of uncovering diagnostic abuses in the silica litigation, and, absent the fortuitous alignment of these factors, litigation based on abusive diagnostic practices might have continued.

The proceedings in front of Judge Jack offer an opportunity to identify the actions that led to the uncovering of abusive diagnostic practices. We do not suggest that the experience with silica is necessarily relevant to all mass personal-injury litigation. However, reviewing the experience of silica litigation can help suggest changes that should be considered to increase the likelihood that similar diagnostic practices will be uncovered should they occur in future mass torts or prevented from occurring in the first place.

In this report, we describe the proceedings in the court of Judge Jack. We then identify factors that worked in favor of as well as against exposing the diagnostic abuses. Our review suggests several areas in which changes to the tort system may increase the likelihood that similar practices would be uncovered in the future. However, the scope of this study does not allow us to recommend the implementation of specific changes in legal practices or procedures. Rather, we identify the types of changes that are worthy of further consideration and analysis.

The remainder of this chapter provides background on the health effects of exposure to silica dust and on the history of silica-related ligation up to the aggregation of cases in front of Judge Jack. We then describe the research methods used in our analysis and outline the report's organization.

Health Effects of Silica Exposure

Crystalline silica in the form of quartz, the second-most abundant mineral on earth, is usually harmless. However, when it is in the form of very small particles that can reach deep inside the lungs (respirable silica), it can cause silicosis.[1] Silicosis is an incurable disease that results from scarring of the lungs. Exposure to respirable silica can also result in lung cancer and chronic obstructive pulmonary disease. It can increase susceptibility to tuberculosis and other pulmonary infections and has been associated with autoimmune diseases. Workers in many industries, including mining, quarrying, construction, glass, cement, abrasives, ceramics, and iron and steel mills, can be exposed to silica.

As documented in Appendix A, review of the available scientific literature suggests that death and disease due to silica exposure in the workplace have declined substantially in the past 40 years.[2] The official count of silicosis-related deaths in the United States between 1968 and 2003 stands at 7,642. Over that period, the annual count has dropped sixfold, from 1,065 silicosis-related deaths in 1968 to 179 silicosis-related deaths in 2003. There is no accurate measure of how many current and former workers have silicosis. Based on the methods outlined in Appendix A, we estimate that there were between 14,000 and 28,000 new silicosis cases in 1968. The estimated number of new silicosis cases declined between 1968 and 2003, and, by 2003, we estimate that there were between 2,400 and 4,700 new silicosis cases annually.

---

1 Respirable silica can be produced when silica-containing materials are shattered or pulverized in the workplace. Respirable silica also occurs naturally. Note that not all silica dust is respirable silica. Some or all of the particles in a given sample of silica dust may be insufficiently small to reach deep inside the lungs.

2 Appendix A describes the types of injuries associated with silica exposure and reviews estimates of the number of workers exposed to silica dust. It presents trends in the number of deaths due to silica in the past 40 years and updates previous research to develop projections of the number of new silicosis cases annually.

The Rise and Fall of Silica Litigation

The compensation of workers who claim to have been injured because of exposure to silica dust has been the subject of major public policy and legal debates in the past 100 years. In the first decades of the 20th century, silica-related injuries were thought inappropriate for inclusion in early workers' compensation programs because of the potentially long latency period of the disease and the potential difficulty of determining which employer was responsible for the exposure. A spurt of litigation in the 1930s, however, led many state legislatures to conclude that workers' compensation was preferable to tort for silica injuries. Tort litigation over silica-related injuries consequently disappeared for more than three decades. Silica litigation began to reemerge in the 1970s. Small numbers of tort cases began to appear in the 1970s, increasing gradually through the second half of the 1990s. Appendix B reviews the evolution of the litigation through the 1990s and identifies the factors that led to a resurgence of silica litigation in the 1970s.

The character of silica litigation changed in the late 1990s. Following the experience of asbestos litigation, some plaintiffs' law firms began to conduct mass screenings for silica-related diseases.[3] In addition, some law firms also rescreened previous asbestos clients for the possibility that they may be suffering from silicosis or mixed-dust pneumoconiosis. These screenings produced medical reports finding silicosis in many of the screened persons. As a result, there was a huge upswing in silicosis claims beginning in 2001—most filed in Mississippi and Texas, states that had earlier attracted a substantial share of asbestos litigation.[4]

U.S. Silica, one of the nation's largest silica providers, reported a dramatic increase in claims against it in the early 2000s (see Figure 1.1). The number of claims jumped to 1,356 in 2001, more than twice the annual average observed in the second half of the 1990s, before soaring to 5,277 in 2002 and 19,865 in 2003.

Nearly two-thirds of the claims filed against U.S. Silica between 2001 and 2003 were filed in Mississippi state courts, and most of the remaining were filed in Texas state courts. During this period, Mississippi had liberal joinder provisions that allowed plaintiffs to file lawsuits in Mississippi even if their connection to the state was quite tangential.

The defendants in a number of the claims sought to remove them to federal court. In 2003, claims by more than 10,000 silica plaintiffs naming 250 defendants were aggregated under Multidistrict Litigation 1553 (MDL 1553) in the Southern District

[3] In principle, mass screenings have the potential to identify undiagnosed sufferers of silicosis (and other diseases) and to ensure that they receive proper medical treatment and appropriate prophylactic measures to avoid further injury to their lungs. As is described later, there is evidence that, in the case of silica, at least some screenings did a very poor job of determining whether those screened were suffering silica-related injuries.

[4] Between 1998 and 2000, 18 and 19 percent of all asbestos claims filed in state courts were filed in Mississippi and Texas, respectively (Carroll et al., 2005, p. 62).

of Texas before U.S. District Court Judge Janis Graham Jack to determine whether the federal courts had jurisdiction based on diversity (*In re Silica Products Liability Litigation*, 398 F. Supp. 2d 563, 566).[5] In making this determination, however, Judge Jack took the unusual step of conducting a *Daubert* hearing[6] after she became increasingly suspicious of the basis for the lawsuits.

In June 2005, Judge Jack issued an order that questioned the validity of virtually every claim within the multidistrict litigation. The court criticized the procedures used by the doctors who diagnosed the vast majority of the plaintiffs and ordered sanctions against plaintiffs' attorneys, finding that their behavior had been unreasonable and vexatious. Silica litigation plummeted following Judge Jack's order. Plaintiffs' firms voluntarily dismissed the bulk of the silica claims remanded to state courts ("Law Firms Won't Be Sanctioned Over Silica Screenings," 2007). New filings against U.S. Silica fell to 1,900 claims in 2005 and to 227 claims in 2006 (see Figure 1.1). Only 15 claims were filed against U.S. Silica in the first half of 2007.

Research Approach

We reviewed the proceeding before Judge Jack to identify the actions that led to the uncovering of abusive diagnostic practices. As noted earlier, we do not suggest that the experience with silica is necessarily relevant to all mass personal-injury litigation. However, the experience of silica litigation can suggest changes that should be considered to increase the likelihood that similar diagnostic practices will be uncovered in the future or prevented from occurring in the first place. We approached this analysis in a number of ways.

First, we drew on data and knowledge from previous RAND Institute for Civil Justice research on asbestos and other mass toxic tort litigation to establish historical and interpretative contexts for the silica multidistrict litigation.[7]

Second, we reviewed the proceedings before Judge Jack in detail. We reviewed the transcripts of the depositions of the diagnosing doctors and the transcript of the *Daubert* hearing.

---

[5] Plaintiffs' attorneys bundled multiple claims in the cases filed in Texas and Mississippi state courts. The roughly 10,000 claims removed to federal court were grouped in 111 cases. Of the 111 cases in the multidistrict litigation, 107 were originally filed in Mississippi state courts. The purpose of multidistrict litigation is to provide common pretrial processing for a set of similar claims. In general, removal from state to federal court is permitted only when there is "complete" diversity of parties—that is, when the plaintiffs are all citizens of states other than that of the defendants.

[6] In a *Daubert* hearing, the judge hears evidence on the reliability and relevance of expert evidence that parties desire to introduce into a case. The standards for review were initially set forth by the U.S. Supreme Court in *Daubert v. Merriell Dow Pharms.* in 1993 (509 U.S. 579) and expanded upon in later decisions.

[7] See Carroll et al. (2005) and other studies cited there.

Figure 1.1
Claims Against U.S. Silica, 1975–2007

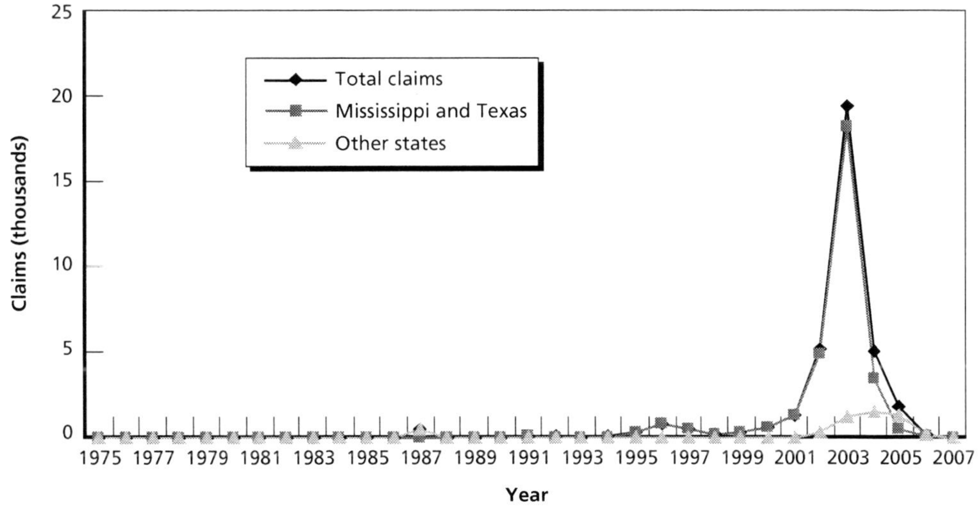

SOURCE: U.S. Silica (2007).
NOTE: Claim figures for 2007 run through June 2007.
RAND *TR774-1.1*

Third, we obtained confidential data from a major silica defendant on the number of claims by year and state going back to 1975 and on sand shipments by year and state back to 1992. We specified the data we sought and conducted sufficient investigation to assure ourselves that the data provided to us were reliable.

Fourth, we interviewed 43 individuals who have been involved in various aspects of silica litigation, to develop a broad view of how the silica multidistrict-litigation process led to the identification of questionable diagnostic practices in the litigation. We interviewed three plaintiffs' attorneys, 17 defense attorneys, and one judge who had been involved in the litigation. We also interviewed a senior representative at eight major silica defendants and ten insurers that have covered major silica defendants. Finally, we interviewed three academics who have conducted extensive analyses of silica litigation and one federal congressional staff member who has collected information for congresspersons concerned with various aspects of silica litigation.

Interviews were conducted on a confidential basis in person or by telephone and were guided by an interview guide developed by the research team. The interview guide outlined the topics to be covered during the discussion, rather than a specific set of questions.

In parallel with the data-collection activities and interviews, we reviewed the development and evolution of silica litigation to understand how the mass litigation that emerged in the late 1990s differed from what had been the trends and patterns in silica litigation previously.

Finally, we reviewed the epidemiology of the health effects associated with silica exposure.

Organization of This Report

Chapter Two describes the proceedings before Judge Jack that led to the discovery of gross deficiencies in the medical diagnoses of silica-related injuries. Chapter Three examines the key factors that enabled these practices to be uncovered. Chapter Four suggests areas in which practitioners and policymakers should consider modifications to the tort system that could deter or expose such behavior in the future. Appendix A reviews the epidemiology of health effects associated with exposure to silica, and Appendix B reviews the evolution of the litigation through the 1990s.

CHAPTER TWO

The Exposure of Diagnostic Abuses in Silica Litigation

A sequence of events occurred in Judge Jack's court that led to the exposure of gross deficiencies in the diagnoses underlying the silica claims in front of her. While the abuses were exposed through court decisions, the decisions were the result of the way in which defendants presented information to the court and the way in which the court responded. This chapter highlights the key developments in the proceedings.

In re Silica Products Liability Litigation

The roughly 10,000 claims were transferred to Judge Jack in 2003. Judge Jack initiated proceedings to determine whether the federal courts had diversity jurisdiction. The legal proceedings, however, expanded well beyond what is usually involved in making this determination, after Judge Jack became increasingly suspicious of the validity of the lawsuits.

Fact Sheets

In January 2004, Judge Jack issued a discovery order to determine subject-matter jurisdiction: whether the defendants' efforts to remove the cases from state court to federal courts could be sustained on the basis of diversity jurisdiction. Uncommonly, the discovery order required the submission of sworn fact sheets to "develop the factual basis for the claims of each plaintiff" (Order No. 29, p. 20). Each fact sheet was required to specify the plaintiff's diagnosis and all pertinent medical and diagnostic information, as well as the results of B-reads of chest x-rays.[1] Plaintiffs were instructed to provide a 20-year history of pneumoconiosis and to identify the treating physician for each plaintiff. The fact sheet for each plaintiff was to be submitted by April 5, 2004. If a plaintiff failed to do so, his or her claim would be dismissed.

[1] B-reads are done by physicians who have been certified through the B-reader program of the National Institute for Occupational Safety and Health (NIOSH). The program certifies that doctors are trained to interpret pulmonary x-rays using the International Labour Organization (ILO) International Classification of Radiographs of Pneumoconiosis.

Judge Jack and the defense attorneys reviewed the fact sheets provided by plaintiffs and soon identified several patterns in the information that they thought suspicious.

First, the fact sheets showed that, in almost all the cases, the plaintiff's claim was not based on a diagnosis provided by the plaintiff's treating physician but rather by doctors affiliated with a handful of law firms and mobile x-ray screening companies. In virtually every case, the diagnosing doctors were "not the Plaintiffs' treating physicians, did not work in the same city or even state as the Plaintiffs, and did not otherwise have any obvious connection to the Plaintiffs" (Order No. 29, p. 31).

Second, although almost all the plaintiffs had different treating physicians, a very small number of B-readers accounted for almost all the plaintiffs' B-reads and diagnoses. More than 9,000 plaintiffs who submitted fact sheets had listed approximately 8,000 different treating physicians but had been diagnosed with silicosis by only 12 doctors (Order No. 29, p. 30).

The defense attorneys found familiar the names of the B-readers who had provided the diagnosis for the vast majority of the plaintiffs. Many of the defense firms had been retained because they had been involved in asbestos litigation and had considerable expertise in the issues related to injuries resulting from inhaling dust in the workplace. Because of their familiarity with asbestos litigation, they recognized that some of the B-readers who figured prominently in the silica multidistrict litigation had been involved in asbestos litigation.

The defense firms then reviewed the available information on asbestos claimants, using both files they had developed in the course of defending asbestos claims and lists of asbestos claimants obtained from other sources, such as court records. They soon discovered that a substantial fraction of the plaintiffs in the silica multidistrict litigation had earlier filed claims for asbestos-related injuries.

The Doctors' Depositions

The defendants sought discovery from nine of the diagnosing doctors and three of the x-ray screening companies. Two of the screening companies contested the defendants' discovery subpoenas in the U.S. District Court for the Southern District of Mississippi. Plaintiffs filed motions in Judge Jack's court to quash the discovery subpoenas issued to the other screening company and the nine doctors. The plaintiffs argued that the discovery subpoenas should be quashed because each of the doctors was a plaintiffs' consulting expert. However, four days after the motions to quash were filed with Judge Jack, and before the defendants responded or the court ruled, the defendants succeeded in deposing one of the diagnosing doctors.

The defendants deposed George Martindale on October 29, 2004. Martindale testified that he was not a plaintiffs' expert and had specifically refused the plaintiffs' lawyers' request that he serve as their expert.

The fact sheets submitted by 3,617 plaintiffs listed Martindale as the diagnosing doctor. The 3,617 diagnoses attributed to Martindale were done in 48 days—

approximately 75 per day (Order No. 29, p. 35). Each report that he filed contained exactly the same diagnosis language:

> On the basis of the medical history review, which is inclusive of a significant occupational exposure to silica dust, physical exam and the chest radiograph, the diagnosis of silicosis is established within a reasonable degree of medical certainty. (Order No. 29, p. 32)

Despite this language, during this deposition, Martindale testified that he

- did not diagnose any plaintiff
- never spoke with a single plaintiff
- did not know the criteria for diagnosing silicosis.

Martindale then withdrew all of the alleged diagnoses, claiming that he assumed that he was simply confirming a diagnosis made by each plaintiff's personal physician, although no such diagnoses were ever made.

During his deposition, it was revealed that "All of Dr. Martindale's reports and B-reads were works hired by N&M, Inc., the screening medical company that orchestrated the majority of silicosis diagnoses for plaintiffs in this MDL" (Order No. 29, p. 35). Martindale testified that Heath Mason, co-owner of N&M, had told him that an abbreviated history, a physical, and a B-read had previously been performed for each plaintiff by a radiologist, Ray Harron (Order No. 29, pp. 35–36). N&M mailed Martindale a packet for each person, containing a chest x-ray in a jacket, a one-page medical history and physical, and an ILO form with the plaintiff's and Martindale's identifying information already filled in.[2] The x-ray jacket had a notation, which Martindale thought had been written by Harron. Martindale would note Harron's B-read for each plaintiff, look at the plaintiff's x-ray, complete the ILO form, and dictate a report. He then mailed the completed form and dictation tape and the other materials that had been sent to him to a transcriptionist specified by N&M. The transcriptionist typed the report, inserting the "diagnosis of silicosis" language. The transcriptionist then sent the typed report to N&M, which stamped them with Martindale's signature. Martindale testified that he had never seen one of his "diagnosing reports."

With Judge Jack's permission, the defendants subsequently deposed two other doctors, Glyn R. Hilburn and Kevin Cooper, who had been listed as the diagnosing doctors on 471 and 255 plaintiff fact sheets, respectively. Both doctors essentially echoed Martindale's testimony. They both testified that they had never diagnosed silicosis and that N&M had inserted the diagnosis-of-silicosis language into their reports without their knowledge. Both doctors recanted their diagnoses.

---

2 The ILO form is used to record the results of a B-read.

Judge Jack expressed concern about Martindale's testimony—particularly his withdrawal of his diagnoses—and concluded that more discovery into the screenings was needed.[3] In February 2005, she issued Order No. 19, which required that every doctor who diagnosed silicosis for any of the plaintiffs and representatives of two of the screening companies attend in person and testify at a *Daubert* hearing.

The *Daubert* Hearings

Judge Jack noted that a *Daubert* hearing was the

> most efficient and effective way to allow the Defendants to depose the doctors (as is their right under the Federal Rules of Civil Procedure), while providing direct court supervision over the proceedings . . ., which seemed advisable in the light of the allegations . . . of misconduct made by both sides. (Order No. 29, p. 42)

The judge also noted that, for two reasons, the court would conduct the hearing before deciding subject-matter jurisdiction. First, the defendants had moved for sanctions, which a court without subject-matter jurisdiction may consider. And, second, one method for determining subject-matter jurisdiction is through the doctrine of improper joinder, which would apply if there was fraud in the pleading of facts (Order No. 29, p. 44).

A representative of each of two medical screening companies, N&M and RTS, testified at the *Daubert* hearing. The two companies hired most of the diagnosing doctors for the multidistrict litigation. N&M identified 6,757 of the plaintiffs; RTS accounted for 1,444 of the plaintiffs. These firms had originally been formed to screen potential asbestos plaintiffs but were asked by plaintiffs' law firms to start screening potential silicosis plaintiffs as well. N&M, which had no medical director, paid Ray Harron $125 per person to follow a three-step process—read an x-ray, perform an abbreviated physical examination, and make a diagnosis. In most cases, an employee provided by a temporary-employment agency would take the exposure history over the telephone. As the court wrote,

> There is no evidence that anyone answering the phones, whether employed by a screening company or a law firm, had any medical training or had been instructed by any medical professional what questions would be appropriate in taking an occupational history. (Order No. 29, p. 68)

---

[3] In her June 30, 2005, order, Judge Jack wrote,

> At the next in-person status conference after Dr. Martindale's deposition, on December 17, 2004, the Court expressed concern about Dr. Martindale's withdrawal of his diagnoses, and thereafter proposed *Daubert* hearings/Court depositions for all of the remaining diagnosing doctors, as well as the screening companies (such [as] N&M) that hired most of them. (Order No. 29, p. 39)

Moreover, N&M was paid by the hiring law firm only for positive diagnoses. Payment was contingent on a positive diagnosis and the potential plaintiff signing with the law firm. Judge Jack characterized N&M strategy as follows: "[T]he emphasis was on attracting as many people as possible to the screenings and creating as many positive diagnoses as possible" (Order No. 29, p. 75). She concluded that, "Overall, N&M—a small Mississippi company operated without medical oversight—managed to generate the diagnoses for approximately 6,757 MDL plaintiffs" (Order No. 29, p. 79). The court also underscored the fact that many of the plaintiffs in the multidistrict litigation had previously been diagnosed with asbestosis—nearly two-thirds of those from N&M screenings.

Perhaps the key witness during the *Daubert* hearing was Ray Harron, who had retired from regular practice in 1995 and subsequently read x-rays and provided diagnostic reports for plaintiffs' lawyers. This work started with asbestosis and eventually shifted to silicosis. One of the first issues addressed was the standards used in Harron's diagnostic reports. Many of the diagnostic reports stated the plaintiff had been diagnosed with silicosis to a "reasonable degree of medical certainty." Harron admitted under oath that the diagnosis he provided was "a legal standard and not a real diagnosis" (Order No. 29, p. 81). He testified that he had not conducted physical exams on any of the plaintiffs nor did he take an exposure history—instead, he relied on forms prepared by plaintiffs' law firms and N&M. In fact, he did not consider other potential causes for lung dysfunction, a fundamental criterion for a diagnosis, because N&M had told him that there was silica exposure (Order No. 29, p. 55).

In essence, Harron only took a quick look at the x-rays and filled out an ILO form. He had nothing to do with preparing the diagnostic reports. In many cases, a typist was left to translate the information on the ILO form into a diagnostic report. Although other diseases could have been responsible for the opacities on the x-ray, the typists (with no medical training) generally interpreted the x-ray reading as consistent with silicosis or asbestosis (Order No. 29, pp. 84–86). As the court writes, "in every one of the approximately 6,350 reports . . . purportedly issued by Dr. Harron, Dr. Harron failed to write, read, or personally sign the actual reports." Harron performed approximately 78 percent of the B-reads for the multidistrict-litigation plaintiffs who submitted diagnoses.

Even more disturbing was the number of former Harron asbestos diagnoses that became silicosis diagnoses for the same plaintiff in silica litigation. Judge Jack wrote,

> In short, when Dr. Harron first examined 1,807 plaintiffs' x-rays for asbestos litigation (virtually all done prior to 2000, when mass silica litigation was just a gleam in a lawyer's eye), he found them all to be consistent only with asbestosis and not with silicosis. But upon re-examining these 1,807 x-rays for silica litigation, Dr. Harron found evidence of silicosis in every case. (Order No. 29, p. 90)

The implausibility of these findings was further underscored by extensive evidence cited by Judge Jack that the co-occurrence of silicosis and asbestosis is extremely rare (Order No. 29, pp. 134–135).

It became clear during the testimony of James Ballard, another of the diagnosing physicians, that similar practices were followed for plaintiffs screened by RTS. He testified that he did not perform physical examinations or take exposure histories for any of the nearly 1,500 B-reads he conducted. Like Harron, he also read a number of x-rays differently depending on what the hiring law firm was looking for—initially asbestosis, then silicosis. Ballard testified that

> a simple statement from the lawyers or RTS that there is exposure history that's consistent with asbestosis [meant] that the lawyers and/or RTS wanted [him] to look for asbestosis. Dr. Ballard acknowledged that this could sway his reading. (Order No. 29, p. 94)

Barry Levy, a physician who diagnosed nearly 1,400 plaintiffs, also testified at the hearing. Levy admitted that

> he did not take occupational or medical histories of any of the plaintiffs; he did not perform the B-reads on any of the plaintiffs; he did not perform the physical examination of any of the plaintiffs; and he did not speak to any of the plaintiffs or their primary care physicians. (Order No. 29, p. 97)

The protocol he set up relied totally on B-reads by other doctors and examinations by other medical professionals—although he stated he was not sure whether the protocol was actually followed. He spent only four minutes on each diagnosis.

Judge Jack's *Daubert* Analysis

Based on this testimony from diagnosing doctors and experts from the occupational and pulmonary health fields, Judge Jack provided a detailed *Daubert* analysis. Her June 2005 opinion began by stating that the number of claims filed in the multidistrict litigation defied all medical knowledge and logic.[4] As Gary Friedman, who is an occupational medicine expert and professor at the University of Texas, had testified, "There simply is no rational medical explanation for the number of alleged diagnoses of silicosis in this MDL" (Order No. 29, p. 116).

Judge Jack suggested two main theories regarding why there had been a spike in silica litigation: (1) claims were filed to beat the tort reforms taking effect in Mississippi in September 2004 and (2) the decline in asbestosis litigation left a network of

[4] The court noted that, in contrast to the huge number of silica filings between 2002 and 2004, the Centers for Disease Control and Prevention had found that both the number of U.S. workers exposed to silica dust and the number of silicosis-related deaths in the United States had steadily declined since 1970 (Order No. 29, p. 10).

plaintiffs' lawyers and screening companies looking for new means of support (Order No. 29, p. 116).[5] With this foundation set, she moved into the analysis. Judge Jack wrote, "In this MDL . . . the issue is whether the actual proffered diagnoses are reliable" (Order No. 29, p. 119). She noted that the answer to this question turns on whether the methodology used by the diagnosing doctors is correct and is applied correctly. To determine reliability, three criteria must be met:

> A diagnosis requires (1) an adequate exposure to silica dust with an appropriate latency period, (2) radiographic evidence of silicosis, and (3) the absence of any good reason to believe that the radiographic findings are the result of some other condition (i.e., a differential diagnosis). (Order No. 29, pp. 120–121)

Judge Jack used these criteria to judge the worthiness of the diagnoses in the multidistrict litigation.

Judge Jack found that the exposure and health histories were taken by people who not only had no medical training but had a financial interest in the outcome of a diagnosis. Medical experts had testified that a diagnosis required a detailed occupational history conducted by a fully trained medical professional. These doctors also made it clear that understanding a suspected silicotic's health background (particularly whether he or she was a smoker) was crucial. Furthermore, most of the histories that were actually taken

> were devoid of meaningful details, such as the duration and intensity of exposure, which are critical to determining whether someone has sufficient exposure, dosage, and latency to support a reliable diagnosis. . . . Instead, the evidence shows that none of the challenged experts took an occupational or exposure history. They all relied upon a history taken by lawyers and clerks with no medical training. (Order No. 29, pp. 122–126)

Based on these findings, Jack held,

> Looking no further than the first criterion, virtually all of the diagnoses fail to satisfy the minimum, medically-acceptable criteria for the diagnosis of silicosis, and therefore, the testimony of the challenged doctors cannot be admissible. . . . (Order No. 29, p. 129)

With regard to the radiographic evidence presented, the single biggest issue that the court addressed was the near sole reliance of the diagnosing doctors on x-rays. As

[5] Civil justice reforms were implemented in Mississippi in 2003 and 2004 (Behrens, Lorber, and Silverman, 2005; Carroll et al., 2005, p. 29). Other factors that may have contributed to the spurt in silica litigation include the federal legislation being considered at the time that would have created a national trust fund for asbestos claims and the increase in asbestos-related bankruptcies (Behrens, Lorber, and Silverman, 2005). Both these factors could lead to reduced asbestos litigation and lower attorney fees.

Judge Jack wrote, "a positive B-read simply does not equal a diagnosis" (Order No. 29, p. 128). Judge Jack also called attention to the fact that the B-readers were told to look for silicosis, a method that does not follow accepted medical practice. She writes, "it is clear that at least some of [the] pressure to produce positives was transferred to the B-readers/diagnosing doctors" (Order No. 29, p. 133).

Turning to the testimony regarding the 6,000 former asbestos plaintiffs who had subsequently been diagnosed with silicosis using the same x-ray, the court concluded,

> The unsound nature of the diagnoses is betrayed not only by the opportunistic transformations of asbestosis reads into silicosis reads, but also by the improbable consistencies among the silicosis reads. . . . [T]he consistencies in profusions [on the x-ray images] defies all statistical logic and all medical and scientific evidence of what happens to the lung when it's exposed to workplace dust. (Order No. 29, p. 135)

In addressing potential differential diagnoses, Judge Jack writes, "In almost all of the MDL cases, the challenged diagnosing doctors simply ignored this final criterion" (Order No. 29, p. 137). The opinion concluded that the failure to address other explanations for x-ray evidence or lung distress was not consistent with generally accepted practice within the occupational medicine industry. Rather than take a thorough history to distinguish silicosis from other possible causes of lung impairments, the differential diagnoses were made by untrained secretarial personnel. Several of the diagnosing doctors argued that there was no time to make a differential diagnosis for each plaintiff. Perhaps reflecting her own clinical experience as a nurse, Judge Jack concludes, "Hordes of plaintiffs have not been thrust upon [the diagnosing doctors] against their will [and] the sheer volume of plaintiffs does not mean that these professionals' obligations toward each plaintiff has been lessened" (Order No. 29, p. 142).

Judge Jack concluded her *Daubert* analysis by agreeing with expert witness Gary Friedman, who testified that the silicosis "epidemic" was "largely the result of misdiagnosis" (Order No. 29, p. 143). The opinion suggested that the plaintiffs failed to meet all three criteria laid out for a successful silicosis diagnoses. Judge Jack concluded,

> Twelve doctors diagnosed all 9,083 plaintiffs. This small cadre of non-treating physicians, financially beholden to lawyers and screening companies rather than to patients, managed to notice a disease missed by approximately 8,000 other physicians—most of whom had the significant advantage of speaking to, examining, and treating the plaintiffs. One possible explanation is the fact that in every case involving a screening company, the diagnoses were essentially manufactured on an assembly line. The steps in the diagnosing process were divided among a number of different people, not all of whom were qualified and none of whom assumed overall responsibility and oversight for the entire process. . . . The people performing the steps were so compartmentalized that often they did not know the others' identities, let alone whether they were qualified and were performing their assigned

> tasks correctly. . . . By dividing the diagnosing process among multiple people . . . no one was able to take full responsibility over the accuracy of the process. This is assembly line diagnosing. And it is an ingenious method of grossly inflating the number of positive diagnoses. (Order No. 29, pp. 144–146)

After completing her *Daubert* analysis, Judge Jack went a step further and discussed the effects of mass overdiagnosing on the civil justice system and national economy. She writes, "Limited judicial resources are consumed weeding out meritless claims, costing the judiciary, costing other litigants whose suits are delayed, and ultimately costing the public, who pays for a judicial system that is supposed to move with some degree of speed and efficiency" (Order No. 29, p. 151). Judge Jack described the cascading effects of litigating meritless claims, ranging from costs to defendant companies to plaintiffs with meritorious claims to the misdiagnosed plaintiffs who may have other serious conditions. Quoting John Parker, who formerly administered NIOSH's B-read program, perhaps the larger issue within the silica litigation arena is that

> a purported diagnosis in someone who doesn't have this disease . . . detracts from the person who has the serious and life-threatening disease. Not only does a false diagnosis detract from the person who has silicosis, but it potentially harms future silicosis prevention. (Order No. 29, p. 153)

Judge Jack's Order No. 29

Judge Jack issued Order No. 29 in June 2005, presenting her rulings on three issues:

- whether federal subject-matter jurisdiction existed in the multidistrict litigation
- whether the diagnosing doctors used sufficiently reliable methodology for their testimony to be admissible
- whether plaintiffs' counsel should be sanctioned for submitting unreliable diagnoses and failing to comply with discovery orders.

Subject-Matter Jurisdiction. Judge Jack concluded that she had subject-matter jurisdiction over only one of the 111 multidistrict litigation cases. She writes, "the removing defendants failed to designate *any* evidence in support of their position that federal subject-matter jurisdiction exists over these cases" (Order No. 29, p. 202). For this reason, the court remanded nearly all of the claims for lack of subject-matter jurisdiction to state courts. Judge Jack concluded,

> In spite of this, the court has included its findings concerning all of the testimony it received, in hopes that the state courts that ultimately must shepherd these cases to their conclusion will not have to re-hear Daubert-type challenges to these doctors and their diagnoses. (Order No. 29, p. 154)

Reliability of Diagnoses. In an exception to her general finding that the court lacked jurisdiction, Judge Jack found that the federal courts had jurisdiction over *Alexander v. Air Liquide America Corp.* (No. 03-533, S.D. Tex., 2005), a case involving 100 plaintiffs that had been filed in a federal court. She also found that the diagnosing doctors in this case relied on inadequate and unreliable occupational, exposure, and medical histories and consequently concluded that the diagnoses and accompanying testimony were inadmissible. Thus, Judge Jack granted the defendants' motion to exclude the testimony and diagnoses of these two doctors.

It should be acknowledged that some of the plaintiffs may have indeed suffered from silicosis. However, Judge Jack concluded that the evidence submitted was inadequate to determine whether any of the plaintiffs did actually suffer from silicosis.

Sanctions Against Plaintiffs' Counsel. The court also considered the defendants' motion for sanctions against the plaintiffs' attorneys under 28 U.S.C. 1927, which "provides that any attorney . . . who so multiplies the proceedings in any case unreasonably and vexatiously may be required by the court to satisfy personally the excess costs, expenses, and attorneys' fees reasonably incurred because of such conduct" (Order No. 29, p. 232). The *Alexander* suit over which the court retained jurisdiction was filed by the O'Quinn Law Firm of Houston, Texas. Judge Jack found that "it should have been apparent to O'Quinn in late-2003 . . . that it was medically implausible for the plaintiffs' silicosis diagnoses to have been accurate" (Order No. 29, p. 234). Despite this fact, O'Quinn maintained the lawsuit even after Martindale admitted that his alleged diagnoses were not true diagnoses. Judge Jack found that O'Quinn's continued prosecution of its claims multiplied the proceedings unreasonably and vexatiously (Order No. 29, p. 236). The opinion described O'Quinn's behavior as part of a larger process to "overwhelm the defendants and the judicial system" (Order No. 29, p. 238). Thus, the court found that

> filing and then persisting in the prosecution of silicosis claims while recklessly disregarding the fact that there is no reliable basis for believing that every plaintiff has silicosis constitutes an unreasonable multiplication of the proceedings. When factoring in the obvious motivation—overwhelming the system to prevent examination of each individual claim and to extract mass settlements—the behavior becomes vexatious as well. Therefore, the court finds that in *Alexander*, O'Quinn has multiplied the proceedings unreasonably and vexatiously, and the firm will be required to satisfy personally the excess costs, expenses, and attorneys' fees reasonably incurred because of such conduct. (Order No. 29, p. 239)

Because she imposed sanctions only on the plaintiffs' attorneys in the case over which she retained jurisdiction, Judge Jack prorated her estimate of the costs of the proceedings and set the fine at $8,250, a small figure compared to the total costs defendants and the courts likely incurred as a result of the abusive diagnostic practices.

The Aftermath of MDL 1553

Silica litigation plummeted following Judge Jack's order. Plaintiffs' firms voluntarily dismissed the bulk of the silica claims remanded to state courts ("Law Firms Won't Be Sanctioned Over Silica Screenings," 2007). As discussed in Chapter One, new filings against U.S. Silica had slowed to a trickle by 2007. Legal reforms enacted in several states during this period likely also contributed to the decline in claims, but Judge Jack's findings were undoubtedly a driving factor in the end of silica as a mass tort.[6]

The impact of the multidistrict litigation also spread to asbestos litigation. In 2005, the Manville Trust, one of the major trusts set up by the courts to pay asbestos claims, announced that it would no longer accept medical reports in support of asbestos claims from most of the doctors and testing facilities behind the diagnoses in the silica multidistrict litigation (Austern, 2005). One of the doctors suspended by Manville, Ray Harron, had submitted documents in support of at least 53,724 of the approximately 680,000 claims that the Manville Trust had received through 2005 (Glater, 2005; Manville Trust, 2007).[7]

The Manville Trust saw a major decline in claims following the Jack decision. Claims submitted to the Manville Trust that did not involve malignant cancers had grown from roughly 10,000 claims per year in the early 1990s to more than 77,000 claims in 2003. In 2004, after Judge Jack initiated the multidistrict litigation proceedings, the number of nonmalignant claims filed with the trust fell to about 10,000 and remained at that rate through the third quarter of 2007 (Manville Trust, 2007). This spike and subsequent decline in claims may be in large part explained by a 2004 change in payment procedures that cut payment to the least serious nonmalignant claims, but the Jack decision likely played a role.[8]

---

[6] For example, Ohio enacted legislation in 2004 (Ohio Rev. Code §2307.85 et seq.) requiring plaintiffs to demonstrate physical impairment using objective medical criteria in order to bring or maintain a silica-related action. The legislation was limited to the question of impairment and did not address the diagnosis of the plaintiff's injury of disease. Silica and asbestos medical criteria laws were enacted in Texas and Florida in 2005 (Behrens and Goldberg, 2006). In addition, as noted previously, Mississippi adopted a number of civil justice system reforms in 2003 and 2004 that would tend to reduce the number of claims (see Behrens, Lorber, and Silverman, 2005; Carroll et al., 2005). Texas likewise adopted reforms during this period that may have contributed to the reduction in claims (Daniels and Martin, 2006–2007). Passage of the medical-criterion legislation and adoption of legal reforms may have been, in some cases, prompted by Judge Jack's findings.

[7] Harron submitted documents in support of at least this many claims. The Manville Trust recorded data on the diagnosing doctor beginning only in the early 2000s, and Harron may have been the diagnosing doctor on earlier claims. According to a trustee of the Manville Trust interviewed for this study, claim audits by the Manville Trust in the late 1990s had raised serious concerns about the reliability of Harron's asbestos diagnoses. However, the Manville Trust declined to cease accepting medical reports from Harron because it feared that it would be sued.

[8] A 2006 *Wall Street Journal* article (Davies, 2006) attributed the recent decline in mass torts, particularly in asbestos and silica, in part to "a federal judge's finding last year that nearly 10,000 claims of lung damage from silica dust 'were manufactured for money.'"

A Mississippi judge subsequently declined motions for sanctions against another plaintiffs' firm in suits that had been remanded to Mississippi court ("Law Firms Won't Be Sanctioned Over Silica Screenings," 2007). In the end, only one of the plaintiffs' firms involved in the silica litigation ended up paying a penalty for their practices during the silica litigation. And the sanction levied against that firm was small.

Conclusion

Judge Jack allowed wide latitude in discovery proceedings and subsequently conducted *Daubert* hearings of the plaintiffs' diagnostic experts and the screening companies that hired them. In June 2005, Judge Jack issued an order questioning the validity of virtually every claim within the multidistrict litigation. The court criticized the procedures used by the doctors who diagnosed the vast majority of the plaintiffs and ordered sanctions against one of the plaintiffs' firms, finding that its behavior had been unreasonable and vexatious.

The findings of Judge Jack have been widely accepted, and, as a result, both the number of pending silica cases and the number of new filings plummeted following Judge Jack's order. The rulings of Judge Jack effectively put an end to silica as a mass tort, at least for the time being. However, the exposure of grossly inadequate diagnostic practices in the mass of claims filed in the early 2000s was by no means guaranteed. In the next chapter, we examine the actions and factors that facilitated the discovery of these practices.

CHAPTER THREE

Factors That Facilitated or Hindered the Exposure of Diagnostic Abuses in Silica Litigation

As described in Chapter Two, Judge Jack uncovered numerous abuses in diagnosing silica-related injuries. The judge's subsequent order, in June 2005, focused national attention on problematic aspects of how silica claims entered and proceeded through the civil justice system. The uncovering of grossly inadequate diagnostic practices was a significant success for the tort system in handling a mass tort. The federal court's actions and the consequences of those actions clearly demonstrate that the tort system has the capacity to identify questionable claims in a mass tort setting.

However, one should not be too satisfied with the performance of the tort system in this regard. First, the abusive diagnostic practices were used in the first place, and considerable time and expense were incurred in exposing them. A more effective system might have deterred such behavior from occurring in the first place. Second, the tort system does not appear to have been nearly so effective in the largest mass tort to date—asbestos litigation. As discussed in Chapter Two, for example, Harron provided a large number of the medical reports underlying the asbestos claims to the Manville Trust, and, while audits conducted by the Manville Trust had raised serious concerns about the reliability of these reports, the trust continued to accept them.[1]

To help improve the tort system moving forward, it is useful to examine what factors contributed to the uncovering of inadequate diagnostic practices in the silica context. Identifying the reasons the system successfully uncovered grossly inadequate diagnostic practices in this setting may help to identify changes that would increase the likelihood of uncovering inadequate diagnostic practices should they be used in other settings.

This chapter identifies the factors that facilitated or hindered the exposure of diagnostic abuses in silica litigation. Strategies and actions by the defense attorneys contributed to the exposure of diagnostic abuses, as did the actions of Judge Jack. Spe-

[1] The tort system did respond in some ways to inadequate diagnostic practices in asbestos litigation before the Jack decision. According to a lawyer interviewed for this study who is very familiar with asbestos litigation, defendants deeply discounted settlement values for claims based on documentation provided by several of the diagnosing doctors later identified in the silica multidistrict litigation.

cial features of the silica litigation also facilitated documentation of diagnostic irregularities, in a manner that prompted court action. We discuss each in turn.

Actions by Defense Attorneys That Facilitated or Hindered the Exposure of Abuses

Three defense actions were particularly important in the chain of events that ultimately led to the discovery of diagnostic abuse: Defense attorneys aggregated cases, challenged diagnoses, and assembled a client base large enough to support the required data gathering and analysis. Decisions of defense attorneys can be influenced or directed by defendants or defendants' insurers, and defense counsel is typically retained by the insurers. As will become clear below, the interests of these three parties are not always well aligned.

Aggregated Cases

As discussed in Chapter One, defense counsel sought to remove cases filed in Mississippi and Texas state courts to federal court. The temporary collection of a large number of cases in one court allowed the assembly of powerful statistical evidence of diagnostic abuses. A single case in which an x-ray is first found to be consistent only with asbestosis and then found to show evidence of silicosis might be attributed to the very rare presence of both diseases in the same person or intrareader variability.[2] However, the co-occurrence of both diseases or intrareader variability become highly improbable explanations for the 1,807 such x-rays read by Harron. The large number of cases in the multidistrict litigation provided the opportunity to develop such convincing evidence and to demonstrate the pervasiveness of the problem.

The assembly of a large number of cases allowed discovery of a number of other damaging facts about the cases. Analysis of the cases showed that a small number of doctors accounted for a huge number of the diagnoses and that some doctors diagnosed very large numbers of cases in a single day. For example, analysis of the database revealed that one doctor diagnosed "cases at an average rate of 75 diagnoses per day," an implausibly large number (Order No. 29, p. 35). Review of a large number of cases also allowed documentation of systematic shortcuts in the diagnosis process—for example, the use of untrained administrative support staff to take medical histories.

Finally, with the aggregation of a substantial number of cases, it made financial sense for defendants to pay for collection of detailed information about the diagnosing doctors, screening facilities, and diagnostic practices. If there were only a small number of cases at issue, there may have been more pressure to settle the claims rather than incur the discovery and legal costs associated with investigating them. Processing of

---

[2] *Intrareader variability* refers to the normal variation in the B-reads done by an individual B-reader.

modest numbers of cases in individual courtrooms across Mississippi and Texas may never have resulted in the thorough examination of diagnostic practices.

While assembling a substantial number of claims in a single court facilitated the discovery of diagnostic irregularities, it was vigorously opposed by some defense firms. According to a number of the lawyers we interviewed, some defense lawyers opposed removal to federal district because they feared that the case might be assigned to a federal district court judge who was plaintiff friendly.[3] Many defense firms were also concerned that discovery in federal district court could result in a "product ID" book that could be used by plaintiffs' attorneys across the country to bring cases.[4] Defense attorneys feared that plaintiffs' attorneys would use such a book to help their clients identify products that were in the workplace and thus tie particular products and defendants to the injuries alleged by a plaintiff. Previous research in the asbestos setting has also found that defendants believe that large-scale aggregation tilts the playing field against them (Carroll et al., 2005, p. 34). A final reason that defendants, as represented by their attorneys, might oppose aggregation is that it dramatically increases the stakes of a single adjudication. Risk-averse defendants and defense attorneys may prefer smaller, separate adjudications for which the stakes are not so large.[5]

In the case of silica litigation, the defense firms in favor of removing the cases to federal court prevailed, but only after extensive discussion among the defendants, insurers, and defense counsel. Had the arguments against removal won out, the abuses in the diagnostic process might never have been discovered.

Challenged Diagnoses

While it might seem like a pedestrian observation, a critical action by the defense attorneys in the silica multidistrict litigation was to challenge the diagnoses. According to defense counsel involved with the silica multidistrict litigation, some defense attorneys did not want to challenge the diagnoses and were opposed to the confrontational tactics of Forman Perry, the lead defense firm.

There are at least four explanations for the reluctance of some defense attorneys to challenge the silica diagnoses. First, challenging diagnoses adds, at least in the short run, to legal costs. Some defendants and their attorneys may have concluded that the cheapest way out of the litigation was to quickly settle claims without challenging diagnoses.

---

[3] The assignment of Bill Clinton appointee Judge Jack to the multidistrict litigation only reinforced their fears.

[4] A product ID book contains pictures of the packaging used by different silica manufacturers, equipment associated with silica use, such as sandblasting hoses and nozzles, and silica-related safety and protective devices used in the workplace.

[5] Variation in the outcomes of separate adjudications may average out to approach the expected value of the loss for silica cases. The outcome in a single large adjudication may be either very positive or very negative for defendants, and a risk-averse defendant would prefer the expected value (see White, 2004, p. 188).

Second, some insurers may have thought it in their financial interest to settle claims against their policyholders rather than challenge diagnoses. Insurance policies often do not limit the amount paid for defense costs but do contain a cap on the amount of indemnity payments. Thus, from an insurer's perspective, it might make financial sense to settle a case and have the settlement count toward the policy limit rather than add to potentially unlimited defense costs.

Third, concerns about reprisals by plaintiffs' attorneys appear to be an important factor in discouraging defense attorneys from challenging diagnoses. A number of the defense attorneys we interviewed expressed concerns that plaintiffs' attorneys would target their clients in future cases if diagnoses were challenged. Plaintiffs' attorneys have some discretion as to which defendants to sue, and they reportedly threatened to focus future cases on "uncooperative" defendants.

Greater attention to fees than to minimizing the long-term cost of the litigation to their clients is a fourth possible explanation for the reluctance of some defense attorneys to challenge diagnoses. One plaintiffs' attorney interviewed for this study recalled multiple instances in which a defense attorney would call and suggest that his client be named in a silica case. Also, according to some of those interviewed, some defense attorneys increase their revenue by churning a case for a while, mediating the case for a while, and then settling. Actively contesting diagnoses, or even trying a case, could threaten an ongoing, stable source of income.

While these explanations provide powerful disincentives for defense attorneys to challenge diagnoses, several factors reduced their effect in the case of silica litigation. First, according to some of the insurers and defendants we interviewed, decades of asbestos litigation had led some insurers and defendants to believe that quickly settling questionable cases was not the best strategy for reducing the ultimate cost of the litigation. Far from reducing the overall litigation burden, some now believed, settling massive number of questionable claims even at low values can increase the number of claims that are filed and the final cost of the litigation. Some insurers and defendants thus resolved to take a longer view and not focus on short-term savings in legal costs.

Second, the fear of retaliation by plaintiffs' attorneys did not have as much bite in silica litigation as in asbestos litigation. Mesothelioma is a virulent cancer whose only known cause is asbestos exposure, and awards in mesothelioma cases are typically substantial. Asbestos attorneys could therefore credibly threaten to try mesothelioma cases against a recalcitrant defendant. Silica litigation, in contrast, lacks a malignant cancer that is uniquely tied to silica exposure and that will almost automatically result in a substantial plaintiff award.[6]

[6] Mesothelioma is a cancer of the lining of the chest or abdomen. Asbestos is the only demonstrated cause of mesothelioma, although some mesothelioma cases have not been traceable to an asbestos exposure. The disease is regarded as inevitably fatal, usually within one or two years of diagnosis (Carroll et al., 2005, p. 12). Mesothelioma claims accounted for approximately 3 percent of all asbestos-related claims from the late 1980s on (Carroll et al., 2005, p. 75). As discussed in Appendix A, studies have shown that the risk of lung cancer increases with

Finally, while the primary concern for some silica defense firms was to maintain a steady billing stream, there were some law firms that aggressively pushed to investigate the veracity of the diagnoses. The defense firms that wanted to aggressively challenge the diagnoses prevailed in the silica multidistrict litigation, but this outcome was by no means certain.

Assembled a Large Database

The leading defense firm in the silica multidistrict litigation built detailed databases of a large number of silica and asbestos claims. These databases were necessary to confirm that a small number of doctors accounted for a large number of diagnoses and to discover that a substantial number of silica plaintiffs had previously filed asbestos claims. Assembling such databases is time consuming and resource intensive. According to this defense firm, two prerequisites were necessary for this effort to succeed. First, a sufficiently large client base was required to amass the financial resources needed to fund the database construction. While, in principle, a large number of defense firms, each representing a limited number of defendants, could have joined to fund a common database-construction effort, substantial transaction costs could have thwarted cooperation. Forman Perry represented a large number of defendants and was able to broadly spread the costs of database construction. Second, according to defense lawyers interviewed for the study, advances in computer software significantly facilitated and perhaps even made possible the assembly of detailed information on a large number of cases.

Actions by Judge Jack That Contributed to Exposing Abuses

Judge Jack took three main actions that greatly increased the likelihood that the diagnostic abuses would be uncovered. We discuss each in this section.

Ordered Early Disclosure of Diagnoses

Judge Jack required plaintiffs to submit fact sheets that identified each plaintiff's diagnosis and all pertinent medical and diagnostic information early in the case, information essential to uncovering diagnostic irregularities (see the discussion of fact sheets in Chapter Two).

Plaintiffs are typically not required to provide a physician's diagnosis until discovery, and, if a case settles before going to trial, a diagnosis may never be provided.[7] Defense efforts to obtain diagnostic information can be time consuming and costly.

---

cumulative exposure to respirable silica. However, there is no known cancer for which there is a high likelihood that the cancer is due to silica exposure and not other causes.

[7] Plaintiffs may also provide medical reports under a precondition set by defendants for settlement talks.

The back and forth between plaintiff and defendant might go as follows: (1) Defendants secure a waiver from the confidentiality requirements of the Health Insurance Portability and Accountability Act (HIPAA) and then file an interrogatory for the name of the doctors; (2) plaintiffs argue that the physician is a consulting expert and not subject to deposition; (3) defendants challenge the plaintiff's claim, and so on. Judge Jack required a diagnosis at the beginning of the case to avoid the cost and delay of the interrogatory process. In doing so, she departed from usual practice and obtained information critical to evaluating the reliability of the silicosis diagnoses.

Judge Jack had previously worked as a nurse, and some people we interviewed attributed her willingness to require medical and diagnostic information to her familiarity with medical practices and procedures. The picture that emerged from our interviews was that Judge Jack was able to rapidly understand and assess arguments by defendants and plaintiffs over medical evidence as well as to identify what additional information was needed to support or refute claims.

Allowed Deposition of Doctors Providing Diagnoses

The defendants sought discovery from nine diagnosing doctors and three x-ray screening companies. Two screening companies contested the defendants' discovery subpoenas themselves, and, as discussed in the proceeding chapter, plaintiffs' attorneys filed motions in Judge Jack's court to quash the discovery subpoenas issued to the third screening company and the nine doctors. The plaintiffs' attorneys argued that the discovery subpoenas should be quashed because each of the doctors was a consulting and not a testifying expert, because the requests were burdensome, and because of HIPAA patient-confidentiality concerns.

Judge Jack rejected all these arguments and allowed the diagnosing doctors to be deposed. She allowed the defense to question doctors across the entire spectrum of plaintiffs, and, moreover, she directed the diagnosing doctors and screening firms to testify in her presence in the form of a *Daubert* hearing. Leading defense attorneys interviewed for this study commented that the latitude to question doctors across all the plaintiffs in the multidistrict litigation and the opportunity to depose the diagnosing doctors in front of a judge were unprecedented. According to defense attorneys, conducting depositions in front of Judge Jack (as opposed to only with counsel present) reduced the number of plaintiff objections and resulted in more-direct answers. Judge Jack also actively participated in the cross-examination and heard firsthand about the diagnostic practices underlying the claims.

Actively Managed the Case

Judge Jack actively managed the case. She called for early disclosure of diagnoses, required the doctors to be deposed in her presence, and held a monthly status conference with opposing counsel. Her active involvement in the case contrasted with practices that judges sometimes employ when faced with mass or complex litigation.

According to some of those interviewed, it is not uncommon for judges to simply allow cases to churn for a few years in the hope that many will settle. To reduce their large dockets, judges may also push for cases to settle with little investigation of the merits of the underlying claim. Judge Jack took neither of these approaches.

Special Features of Silica Litigation That Contributed to Exposing Abuses

Beyond the actions of defense attorneys and Judge Jack, several features of the litigation itself contributed to the discovery of unreliable diagnostic practices. These features include the preexistence of litigation in a closely related area (asbestos), the absence of a terminal cancer that is clearly linked to silica, and a large number of cases.

Prior Asbestos Litigation

Some of the most damaging pieces of evidence against the plaintiffs were Ray Harron's multiple reads of the same x-ray. While there were several other abuses in the diagnosing process that skillful defense attorneys could exploit to their advantage, such a smoking gun raised the credibility of defense arguments. Prior asbestos claims by silica plaintiffs made such a comparison possible. In addition, many of the doctors and screening companies involved in the silica litigation were active in asbestos litigation. The silica defense attorneys were familiar with their involvement in asbestos and suspicious of their practices. Their familiarity with the experts might have prompted the defense to contest the diagnoses more rapidly and aggressively than they would have otherwise. Indeed, had the plaintiffs' attorneys relied on different doctors and screening firms, the outcome of the silica litigation might have been much different even if the underlying diagnoses had been similarly inadequate.

Lack of a Terminal Cancer Uniquely Associated with Silica

As mentioned already, the absence of a terminal cancer uniquely tied to silica exposure reduced defendant concerns about cases coming to trial or about plaintiffs' attorneys' threats to target defendants who did not settle. It seems reasonable to expect that defendants would be more likely to challenge diagnosis and refuse settlement offers in the absence of a terminal cancer that is presumptively due to silica exposure than in the shadow of one.

Large Number of Cases

The large number of cases that had been filed in state courts created the opportunity to assemble sample sizes that provided convincing evidence of grossly inadequate diagnostic practices. The successive examinations of the same x-ray that first found opacities consistent with asbestosis but not with silicosis and then consistent with silicosis would not have been so damning had they occurred in a few cases. The same result for more than 1,800 x-rays was altogether another matter.

The large number of cases drew considerable attention to the litigation and perhaps also increased defense attorneys' resolve to do what they could to avoid silica becoming a mass tort like asbestos. Indeed, if the plaintiffs' attorneys had not pushed so hard to file a large number of cases in a short time, there may well have been a much lower probability that the abuses in the diagnosing process would have been uncovered.

Conclusion

The large number of claims in mass torts creates incentives for plaintiffs, defendants, and judges to cut corners in developing and evaluating the expert evidence that underlies the claims. Plaintiffs can attempt to overwhelm defendants with claims to force defendants to settle with little attention paid to merits of the claims. It can be extremely costly for defendants to investigate the merits of a substantial proportion of the claims, and some may conclude that it is cheaper, at least in the short run, to settle. Judges have an incentive to push for rapid settlements that clear their overloaded dockets.

Such situations are ripe for the abuse of expert evidence. While mass misdiagnosis was uncovered in silica litigation, the potential for such abuse in future litigation remains.

In the silica litigation, a number of factors worked in favor of the exposure of diagnostic abuses, but a number of factors also worked against it. In the case of silica, the factors that contributed to the discovery of abuse won out, but such may not be the case in other settings. Chapter Four identifies promising ways to increase the chances that enough factors will align in other settings to prevent or uncover grossly inadequate diagnostic practices.

CHAPTER FOUR

Changes That Could Help Prevent or Expose Diagnostic Abuses in Mass Personal-Injury Litigation

The documentation of widespread diagnostic abuses during the silica multidistrict litigation essentially put an end to the use of these practices in silica litigation. Further, the outcomes of the silica multidistrict litigation rippled through the ongoing asbestos litigation. Judges, lawyers, and experts have learned important lessons from the asbestos and silica experiences—lessons that may lead them to adjust their behavior so that we will never again see mass personal-injury litigation based on abusive diagnostic practices.

But we cannot be sure. The outcome of the multidistrict litigation was the result of a fortunate alignment of a number of different defense strategies, judicial actions, and features of the silica litigation itself. No one planned for them to come together as they did, and the tort system does not provide an environment that guarantees that sufficient factors will come together in other settings. For example, had there been a different judge, had the diagnosing doctors not been previously involved in asbestos litigation, or had the plaintiffs not filed so many cases in a short period, the grossly inadequate diagnoses may never have been uncovered. It is entirely plausible that such a fortuitous combination of factors will fail to arise in a future mass litigation built on abusive practices.

The experience with silica litigation generates insights into changes in legal procedure and practice that have the potential to increase the likelihood that abusive diagnostic practices will be uncovered in future mass personal-injury litigation and to improve the quality of the medical diagnoses that are introduced in the first place.[1] If policymakers and practitioners believe that further improvements to the legal system in this area are needed, the pros and cons of these changes should be carefully evaluated.

In this concluding chapter, we summarize the potentially promising changes. We do not recommend the implementation of specific changes here; the full evaluation of implementable reforms is well beyond the scope of this study. Rather, we identify changes that merit further consideration. Because the suggestions are based primarily on a review of one type of litigation, an examination of experiences in other types

---

1 It may be that reforms aimed at reducing diagnostic abuses in individual cases may also be worthy of consideration. However, this study focuses on abuse of diagnostic practices in mass personal-injury litigation.

of litigation would provide increased confidence about whether the benefits of change would outweigh their monetary and other costs for mass personal-injury litigation more generally. In addition, many of the changes we suggest for consideration raise important legal issues that should be more thoroughly explored. There may be need for modifications in the law and the rules of civil procedure at both the federal and state levels, and any changes might raise a variety of complex issues. Further, it is important that the impact of potential changes on the ability of truly injured parties to pursue remedies in the civil justice system be considered.

Several of the proposed changes could be triggered once a sufficient number of cases had been filed, and a mechanism would have to be developed to ascertain whether the appropriate threshold had been met. Defendants might be required to report the number of claims arising out of exposure to the same substance or event to a specified organization or agency, such as the state supreme court or a special master, once the number of claims filed against them exceeded a specified threshold. Or plaintiffs' attorneys might be required to report, to some agency or organization, the number of similar claims they have filed.

We first discuss changes that focus on court procedures and practices. We then turn to changes aimed at influencing the behavior of plaintiff and defense lawyers.[2]

Changes in Judicial Practices and Procedures

Many with whom we spoke emphasized the importance of Judge Jack's training as a nurse in uncovering the diagnostic abuses. We take as axiomatic that the outcomes of the tort system should not rely on the background, training, and idiosyncratic practices of a particular judge.[3] The following changes could create conditions that would increase the likelihood that abuses in diagnostic practices in mass personal-injury litigation would be routinely uncovered regardless of the judge assigned to the case.

Require Diagnosis to Be Provided with Relevant Medical Records at Time of Case Filing Once Litigation Has Achieved Sufficient Size

Requiring disclosure of the diagnosis, the identity of the diagnosing physician, and relevant medical records up front would help ensure adherence to defensible diagnostic practices and allow defendants to more rapidly evaluate claims.

---

[2] Reforms that affect medical experts directly, such as increased oversight boards, might also be considered. However, our focus is on the practices of judges and lawyers.

[3] The idea that the application of the law should not depend on the particular individual administering the law has a long history in Anglo-American legal thought. For example, this principle was expressed in the Massachusetts Constitution by John Adams in 1780, when he wrote that the constitution existed to guarantee "a government of laws and not of men" (Massachusetts Constitution, Art. 30, 1780).

Disclosing the identity of the diagnosing physician would also make it impossible for plaintiffs to broadly shield all of their experts from deposition. Plaintiffs' attorneys often contest deposition of an expert by arguing that the expert is a consulting expert and would not testify in a particular case. Once identified, the diagnosing doctor would be eligible for deposition. In sum, any doctor who is the source of a diagnosis on which the claim is based would be subject to deposition.[4]

The diagnosis, the identity of the diagnosing physician, and relevant medical records are already commonly required by the *Lone Pine* orders that are *sometimes* used for case-management purposes by judges in mass torts.[5] Typically, these orders require the plaintiff to produce prima facie evidence of injuries to avoid summary judgment. The change recommended here would in effect require *Lone Pine* filings in a particular type of litigation once the number of cases of that type has grown sufficiently large.

Providing a diagnosis at the time of filing does not mean that the diagnosis could not be changed as new facts develop during the course of the litigation. Parties would retain the ability to amend their claims over the course of the litigation. For example, the injury or disease may progress over the course of the ligation, and plaintiffs would be allowed to develop additional support for their claims. Or, new facts may come out during the discovery process that strengthen a plaintiff's claim in some fashion. We do not suggest that any initial diagnosis be binding.

Require Parties Early to Present Evidence on Appropriate Diagnostic Practices and Whether They Were Followed

Diagnoses should be based on reasonable medical standards or consistent with accepted medical practice, and, once litigation has reached sufficient scale, it would be beneficial for courts to routinely require that these standards and practices be identified early on in the case. Such a determination could be accomplished using briefs submitted by defense and plaintiffs' lawyers or through hearings in front of the court. At the same time diagnostic standards are identified, the court could also require plaintiffs to demonstrate that these practices were followed in the cases under consideration.[6] If a substantial number of claims are based on diagnosis from a particular doctor, the court

---

[4] Consulting experts would still be shielded from deposition as long as they do not provide a diagnosis or testify.

[5] *Lone Pine* orders take their name from *Lore v. Lone Pine Corp.* (1986 N.J. Super. LEXIS 1626, 1986). In that case, the court ordered the plaintiff to submit documentation regarding each plaintiff's exposure to toxic substances—reports of physicians who provided treatment or diagnoses, along with other basic information relevant to the claim. While somewhat controversial, depending on the specific requirements of the order, *Lone Pine* orders have been used by many courts. See, e.g., *Acuna v. Brown and Root Inc.* (200 F.3d 335, 5th Cir., 2000).

[6] Defendants or the court can currently challenge evidence or particular experts and request *Daubert* or *Frye* hearings. (The *Frye* standard for assessing the admissibility of expert evidence predates the *Daubert* standard and remains in use in some state courts. See *Frye v. United States*, 54 App. D.C. 46, December 3, 1923; Dixon and Gill, 2001.) This recommendation encourages courts hearing mass personal-injury litigation to routinely identify appropriate diagnostic practices and confirm that they were followed.

could consider conducting a hearing on the training of the doctor, whether the doctor is connected to screening facilities, and the procedures followed in his or her practice.

Augment Guidance for Multidistrict Litigation Judges

The parties we formally interviewed and others with whom we spoke over the course of the study generally agreed that the outcome of the proceedings would have probably been very different had Judge Jack not been as proactive as she was. None of those with whom we spoke suggested that the outcome of the silica multidistrict litigation was inappropriate. There was general agreement that the proceedings uncovered highly questionable diagnostic practices and brought an end to an abusive mass litigation.

However, some of those with whom we talked expressed significant reservations regarding the appropriateness of Judge Jack's proactivity. In brief, some people argued that the appropriate role of the judiciary is to apply the law to arguments put forth by the participants in a dispute. In the case of the multidistrict litigation, they felt that Judge Jack stepped outside her appropriate role when she required the plaintiffs to submit fact sheets regarding details of their claims, allowed depositions of the doctors, and held a *Daubert* hearing to probe the procedures used to develop the diagnoses, when the only matter before her was a motion for removal. They felt that the appropriate judicial role in these proceedings should have been limited to examination of the bases for removal of the claims to the federal court and that her actions went well beyond that.

Others thought that her activities were highly appropriate. They argued that she had good reason to question the validity of the diagnoses and that, consequently, her examinations of the medical procedures used to arrive at the diagnoses were appropriate.

These differing perspectives suggest the need to augment guidance for federal and state judges on how they should handle mass personal-injury torts. For example, it may be appropriate to enhance the Federal Judicial Center's (2004) *Manual for Complex Litigation, Fourth,* to provide an assessment of which types of judicial practices have been effective in mass personal-injury litigation and which have not. The manual might identify a set of recommended practices for mass personal-injury cases.

Enhance Mechanisms for Aggregating Information Across Claims for Pretrial Purposes

The silica multidistrict litigation shows how important jointly evaluating a large sample of claims can be in assessing the practices used to diagnose injuries. Aggregating information across claims can also increase the likelihood that the parties involved in the litigation will be able to assemble the financial resources needed to systematically assess the evidence. Procedures exist for aggregating claims for pretrial purposes, such as discovery and evaluation of the evidence, but they have important limitations.[7] For example, cases filed and remaining in different state courts cannot be aggregated across states or combined with cases in federal court (Federal Judicial Center, 2004, p. 377). State cases must meet federal jurisdictional requirements before they can be removed to federal courts and potentially aggregated. The fact that Judge Jack ultimately determined that she did not have jurisdiction over nearly all of the silica claims brought before her illustrates the challenges of aggregating claims.

Policymakers should explore the pros and cons of changes that would facilitate the aggregation of claims in mass personal-injury litigation for pretrial purposes. Next, we suggest a few possibilities that warrant further consideration.

Create an Infrastructure for Voluntary Coordination Between State and Federal Judges. Federal and state court judges frequently cooperate informally to coordinate discovery and pretrial proceedings in mass personal-injury cases (Federal Judicial Center, 2004, p. 377).[8] However, these efforts are ad hoc and must largely be undertaken from the ground up for each new type of litigation. Thought should be given to how to strengthen institutional mechanisms for facilitating voluntary coordination between state and federal judges. For example, an office might be established that is charged with facilitating communication and cooperation between state and federal judges or between state-court judges in mass tort cases. Such an office might include staff to whom judges would routinely turn for special masters who could coordinate discovery in mass torts.

Create a Mechanism That Would Allow Federal Courts to Aggregate Claims in State Courts for the Purpose of Developing Information About the Cases. The previous suggestion relies on voluntary cooperation between state and federal judges. However, such cooperation may not always be forthcoming, and policymakers and practitioners should consider mechanisms that would require mass torts to be gathered in federal court for the purpose of developing information about the cases. The federal court would not need to have any authority to make decisions that constrained the authority of the state courts from which the cases came. Rather, much as Judge Jack did, the federal court would assemble information that would be useful when the cases returned to state court. The federal court would need to be given only the powers necessary to collect and synthesize information about the cases, such as the power to

---

[7] Aggregation of mass tort cases in federal courts can occur in a number of different ways. Cases in a federal district can be assigned to a single judge in that district and consolidated for pretrial or trial purposes under Federal Rule of Civil Procedure 42 (F.R.C.P. 42). As in the silica cases before Judge Jack, cases filed in different federal districts can be transferred for coordinated or consolidated treatment by a single judge under the multidistrict-litigation rule. Cases can also be certified as class actions for litigation or settlement purposes (Federal Judicial Center, 2004, pp. 355–356).

[8] For example, according to the Federal Judicial Center (2004, p. 235), "In the silicone gel breast implant and diet drug litigations, state and federal judges created [a] working relationship that come close to achieving a comprehensive approach to state-federal cooperation."

issue subpoenas, hold hearings, and require depositions. The state actions could also continue at the discretion of the state-court judge while the federal court was developing information about the cases.

A number of very difficult issues would have to be addressed in evaluating the feasibility and desirability of such a proposal. For example, decisions would need to be made on whether the Federal Rules of Evidence or state evidentiary rules would apply and whether the federal court could issue evidentiary findings—for example, on whether the evidence passes the *Daubert* test. Thought would have to be given to how the federal court would enforce court orders. In the standard setting, a judge can dismiss a case if the required information is not provided; in contrast, the judge here would not have the power to dismiss cases. The court could, in principle, use its power to find a party in contempt, but the appropriateness of such an action in this situation would need to be evaluated.

There are many potential drawbacks to expanding the jurisdiction of federal courts to allow aggregation of state court claims for the purpose of developing information. However, as illustrated by the silica experience, the potential advantage of assembling a large number of cases for analysis is substantial. Given the current limitations on aggregating claims spread across courts in multiple states, what some might consider a radical change should nevertheless be explored.

Facilitate Consolidation of Cases Already in Federal Court. The multidistrict litigation process used to consolidate actions pending in multiple federal district courts appears to have worked effectively in silica litigation. It also appears to have worked effectively in asbestos litigation, given that all asbestos cases filed in the federal courts were transferred to Judge Charles Weiner of the Eastern District of Pennsylvania for pretrial management (Carroll et al., 2005, p. 28). However, the statute that permits and governs consolidation of actions pending in multiple federal districts, 28 U.S.C. §1407, allows the federal judicial panel on multidistrict litigation considerable discretion in the decision on whether to consolidate claims.[9] Thus, some uncertainty remains as to whether future mass torts spread across multiple federal courts will be consolidated.

Two reforms may be possible to facilitate appropriate consolidation. The first is to ensure that the judicial panel on multidistrict litigation is aware of cases for which multidistrict litigation may be appropriate. Creating some sort of informational infrastructure to alert the panel of mass tort litigation could assist the panel in wisely exercising its jurisdiction in appropriate cases.

---

[9] Title 28 U.S.C. §1407 provides that,

> When civil actions involving one or more common questions of fact are pending in different districts, such actions may be transferred to any district for coordinated or consolidated pretrial proceedings. Such transfers shall be made by the judicial panel on multidistrict litigation authorized by this section upon its determination that transfers for such proceedings will be for the convenience of the parties and witnesses and will promote the just and efficient conduct of such actions.

Second, 28 U.S.C. §1407 might be formally amended to include a presumption that mass tort claims that exceed a certain threshold will be consolidated into multidistrict litigation. Such a formal presumption would encourage serious consideration of the creation of multidistrict litigation while still preserving discretion of the panel to reject consolidation when idiosyncratic facts about the litigation indicate that consolidation is not appropriate.

Changes in Practices of the Plaintiffs' and Defense Bars

In Judge Jack's view, the plaintiffs' firm in the case over which she retained jurisdiction unreasonably pursued the silica cases even after it became clear that there was no reliable basis for the claims. She may have had similar views of the behavior of the other plaintiffs' firms involved in the litigation, but she was silent, given that she remanded the cases to state court. While plaintiffs' firms are typically the focus of complaints about diagnostic practices, our investigation of silica litigation found that a number of defense-attorney practices enabled litigation based on inadequate diagnoses.[10] The following suggestions attempt to reduce the prevalence of improper behaviors on both the plaintiff and defense sides.

Consider More-Serious Sanctions for Pursuing Cases Based on Grossly Inadequate Diagnoses

Judge Jack fined one plaintiffs' firm the pro rata share of the excess costs, expenses, and attorneys' fees that defendants incurred for the *Daubert* hearing. However, as described in Chapter Two, the fine was so small that the direct financial consequences for the firm were minor. In addition, subsequent defense motions in Mississippi state courts for sanctions against other plaintiffs' firms failed.

Judge Jack imposed sanctions under 28 U.S.C. §1927, which provides that "[a]ny attorney . . . who so multiplies the proceeding in any case unreasonably and vexatiously may be required by the court to satisfy personally the excess cost, expenses, and attorneys' fees reasonably incurred because of such conduct." In contrast to Section 1927, F.R.C.P. 11 allows sanctions that would deter improper attorney conduct, thus allowing penalties greater than the direct cost of the conduct.[11]

---

[10] Several of the plaintiffs' attorneys we interviewed were as vocal in their criticism of the diagnostic practices exposed in the silica multidistrict litigation as defense attorneys were. Also, while the silica litigation in front of Judge Jack focused on abuse in medical documentation supporting plaintiffs, there may well be abuse by defense physicians and experts who fail to find injuries despite their existence. This possibility is not addressed in this report but merits further study.

[11] Rule 11 states that, by submitting a representation to the court, an attorney implicitly certifies that,

> to the best of the person's knowledge, information, and belief, formed after an inquiry reasonable under the circumstances: (1) it is not being presented for any improper purpose, such as to harass, cause unnecessary

The imposition of sanctions on a law firm can have significant effects on its reputation and, consequently, on its ability to attract clients, even if the fine is modest. However, to increase the consequences of unreasonably pursuing claims when there is no reliable basis for believing that the plaintiff has suffered injury, judges should routinely consider fines that would deter the behavior rather than just recover excess costs. We have not been able to detail the sanctions available to state-court judges, but such an assessment is warranted to determine whether they have adequate tools to deter improper conduct.

Policymakers might also consider strengthening Rule 11. In particular, the language of the rule was changed in 1993 to make sanctions discretionary rather than mandatory, even when improper litigation has occurred. While this change may have successfully reduced Rule 11 litigation (Yablon, 2004), it also likely reduced its value in deterring misconduct. A return to a less permissive Rule 11 may be appropriate to discourage frivolous litigation.

Pay Closer Attention to the Performance of the Defense Bar

It is not obvious how to deter defense practices that enable litigation based on inadequate diagnostic practices, in part because such practices are difficult to observe. For example, it is difficult to determine that extent to which a defense attorney is simply churning a claim to generate fees with the ultimate goal of settling, without any concerted effort to challenge suspect diagnoses. However, given the importance of the issue, policymakers and practitioners should seriously consider what types of responses might be effective. For example, policymakers and practitioners might consider developing means to chronicle and evaluate defense tactics in mass personal-injury litigation, including defense tactics directed by defendants' insurers. The results could motivate greater attention to ethics issues in law schools and continuing-education courses, as well as in investigations by professional review panels.

Conclusion

Following our review of the silica multidistrict litigation, we have suggested changes in legal procedure and practice that have the potential to improve the tort system's

---

> delay, or needlessly increase the cost of litigation; (2) the claims, defenses, and other legal contentions are warranted by existing law or by a nonfrivolous argument for extending, modifying, or reversing existing law or for establishing new law; (3) the factual contentions have evidentiary support or, if specifically so identified, will likely have evidentiary support after a reasonable opportunity for further investigation or discovery; and (4) the denials of factual contentions are warranted on the evidence or, if specifically so identified, are reasonably based on belief or a lack of information.

Under Rule 11, sanctions are limited "to what suffices to deter repetition of the conduct or comparable conduct by others similarly situated."

ability to prevent and detect abusive diagnostic practices. Before recommendations on implementation can be made, however, further analysis in a number of areas is warranted. First, these suggestions are based on the review of one type of litigation, and a review of experiences in other types of large-scale personal-injury litigation would provide increased confidence that they would be beneficial in mass personal-injury litigation more generally. Second, the monetary costs of any changes should be assessed, as should the potential impact on the ability of truly injured parties to pursue remedies in the civil justice system. Finally, the suggested changes raise a number of difficult procedural and legal issues that need to be addressed.

APPENDIX A

Epidemiology of the Health Effects Associated with Silica Exposure

Silica is the term used to refer to silicon dioxide (SiO_2), a colorless, odorless, noncombustible solid that occurs naturally in both crystalline and noncrystalline forms (NIOSH, 2002). The most common form of crystalline silica is alpha quartz, which can be found in soil and rocks. Noncrystalline (amorphous) silica is a type of silica whose atoms have no special order or geometric pattern. Crystalline silica occurs naturally and can be the direct or indirect product of manufacturing processes. Inhalation of very small silica particles (respirable silica) poses a threat because particles sufficiently small are not filtered out before reaching the lungs.

Workers can be exposed to silica in many industries, including mining, quarrying, construction, glass, cement, abrasives, ceramics, and iron and steel mills (NIOSH, 2002). Silica sand is used in the manufacturing of glass products (including containers, plate and window glass, and fiberglass); molding and core for foundry work; silicon carbide for metallurgical work; fillers for rubber, paints, and putty; ceramics (including bricks, tiles, porcelain, pottery, refractories, and vitreous enamels); and petroleum. Exposure to respirable crystalline silica has also been reported to result from the materials and processes used by dental-laboratory technicians (Rosenman, Pechter, et al., 2004).

In this appendix, we first review how the understanding of silica risks evolved over time and summarize current understanding of the health effects associated with silica exposure. We then provide an overview of the regulations that government agencies have set for exposure to silica dust, followed by estimates of the number of workers currently being exposed to silica, the number of deaths due to silicosis, and the number of new cases of silicosis annually. Estimates of silica exposure, morbidity, and mortality provide insight into the likelihood of litigation moving forward.

Evolution of the Understanding of Silicosis

During the 1800s, workers and doctors alike had accepted dust as one of the causes of what was generally referred to as *consumption*—a progressive wasting away of the body, especially from pulmonary tuberculosis (Hoffman and Forman, 1908).[1] Consumption, also known as "the great white plague," was the single greatest cause of death in Europe and the United States during this period. Consumption was particularly common among foundry workers, hard-rock miners, cutters, potters, buffers, glass workers, and abrasive blasters (Rosner and Markowitz, 1991, p. 14; Dubos and Dubos, 1952 [1987], p. 10).

By the late 19th century, as germ theory came to dominate medical research, dust was no longer thought as important in the etiology of consumption and lung diseases. By this time, there was nearly unanimous concurrence among medical and health professionals that consumption was caused by bacteria rather than by dust (Ransome, 1890, pp. 51–67). While germ theory and the associated revolution in medicine were critical to understanding the etiology of many diseases, it actually hindered the understanding of silicosis and delayed attention to the occupational causes of silicosis (Rosner and Markowitz, 1991, p. 14). Indeed, some hoped that all diseases of the lung could be cured by a vaccine (Gibbes, 1890).

During the first decade of the 1900s, opinion began to change regarding the etiology of consumption. An influential study conducted by a team of British researchers, led by Thomas Oliver, contended that noninfectious causes of lung ailments were more critical than earlier presumed (Oliver, 1902). Among the diseases that were identified was silicosis. Oliver contended that workers with silicosis would be more likely to become infected with tuberculosis. Through this period, however, most U.S. researchers remained committed to the idea that tuberculosis and silicosis were one and the same condition.

In the United States, it was the insurance industry and progressive-era social reformers rather than the medical community that began focusing on silicosis as a separate disease. In particular, a statistician for the Prudential Life Insurance Company, Frederick Hoffman, was interested in this hypothesis because it explained morbidity and mortality rates among industrial workers better than a bacterial theory. The insurance industry was not as institutionally vested in bacterial explanations for disease, and its interests were increasingly deviating from those of medical and public-health professionals. During this period, when the latter professionals discounted industrial causes for lung diseases, Hoffman's work was vital to identifying silicosis as a distinct disease (Rosner and Markowitz, 1991, pp. 24–26; Hoffman and Forman, 1908).[2]

---

[1] Dust was accepted as only one of a myriad of causes of consumption: "Treatment was to be sensitively gauged not to a disease entity but to such distinctive features of the patient as age, gender, ethnicity, socioeconomic position, and moral status, and to attributes of place like climate, topography and population density" (Warner, 1986, p. 58). The understanding of the illness had important social and moral components that may sound odd today.

[2] A statistician at Metropolitan Life Insurance Company, Louis Dublin, also used an important proto-epidemiological approach to occupational diseases (Dublin, 1925, p. 201). Interestingly, some granite workers focused on the danger of the dust even to the point of being willing to strike over the dusty working conditions in the winter, when there was no ventilation (Rosner and Markowitz, 1991, p. 39).

It was not until the beginning of World War I that the foremost public-health journals seriously considered the nonbacterial explanations pushed forward by insurance-industry statisticians and social reformers. By 1920, health professionals had acknowledged that silicosis was a serious lung condition suffered by groups of U.S. workers and that it significantly increased their risk of getting tuberculosis (Rosner and Markowitz, 1991, p. 30; Hayhurst, 1914, p. 10).

Current Understanding of the Health Effects Associated with Silica Exposure

The primary route of exposure for health effects from silica dust is inhalation. According to observations from animal studies, when crystalline silica is deposited in the lungs, it can activate and injure the epithelium and macrophages[3] (IARC, 1997). Crystalline silica can also initiate an inflammation response at the cellular level, the magnitude of which depends on the level of exposure. Following human exposure to crystalline silica, a high proportion of the substance remains in the lungs, possibly resulting in the occurrence of silicosis, chronic obstructive pulmonary disease, emphysema, and lymph-node fibrosis. Human subjects with silicosis demonstrate acute lung inflammation with increased macrophage and lymphocyte activity. Based on animal studies, it has been concluded that tumor development following exposure to crystalline silica results from pronounced chronic inflammation and epithelial proliferation (IARC, 1997).

Silica-Related Diseases

Silicosis. Silicosis is the respiratory disease most commonly associated with exposure to silica. It is a nodular pulmonary fibrosis caused by inhalation of silica particles.[4] There are three types of silicosis:

- chronic silicosis (exposure to low concentrations of silica for ten or more years)
- accelerated silicosis (develops five to ten years after the first exposure to silica)
- acute silicosis (occurs from weeks up to five years after exposure to high concentrations of silica) (American Thoracic Society, 1997; NIOSH, 2002).

The likelihood and severity of silicosis depend on the dose of respirable dust to which one is exposed. Several epidemiological studies of workers exposed to respirable

---

[3] The epithelium is the cellular layer covering all surfaces of the body, both internal and external (Stedman, 1990). In this context, it refers to the lung epithelium. Macrophages are "mononuclear cells which are largely scavengers ingesting dead tissue and degenerated cells" (Stedman, 1990).

[4] Fibrosis is the "formation of fibrous tissue as a reparative or reactive process, as opposed to formation of fibrous tissue as a normal constituent of an organ or tissue" (Stedman, 1990).

silica dust have shown a consistent relationship between the cumulative amount of silica dust inhaled and the development of silicosis. Several studies of occupational cohorts demonstrate this relationship clearly.[5] The development and severity of silicosis also depend on the particle size, the crystalline or noncrystalline nature of the silica, the duration of exposure, and the length of time from first exposure to diagnosis, as well as patient characteristics. Long periods might elapse between exposure to silica and diagnosis of silicosis, meaning that development and progression of the disease might occur after exposure to silica has ceased (Hnizdo and Sluis-Cremer, 1993; Hnizdo and Murray, 1998; Ng, Chan, and Lam, 1987; Kreiss and Zhen, 1996).

Pulmonary Tuberculosis and Other Infections. Persons with silicosis develop pulmonary tuberculosis (TB) at a higher rate than those without silicosis (NIOSH, 2002).[6] It has been hypothesized that, when a worker is exposed to respirable silica dust, the macrophages in the lungs can be overwhelmed by the dust and are, therefore, unable to destroy the bacteria that causes tuberculosis (*Mycobacterium tuberculosis*). Other respiratory infections occurring in workers exposed to silica dust are caused by the nontuberculous mycobacteria (*Mycobacterium kansasii* and *Mycobacterium avium-intracellulare*) or other organisms (*Nocardia asteroids* and *Cryptococcus)* (NIOSH, 1992).

Lung Cancer. Inhaled crystalline silica in the form of quartz or cristobalite has been classified as a human carcinogen by the International Agency for Research on Cancer (IARC) (Wilbourn et al., 1997; IARC, 1997). This conclusion is based on evidence from several epidemiological studies supporting an increased risk of lung cancer following occupational exposure to inhaled crystalline silica.[7] These studies indicate that the risk of lung cancer increases with cumulative exposure to respirable silica, duration of exposure, peak intensity of exposure, presence of radiographically defined silicosis, and length of follow-up time since silicosis diagnosis (NIOSH, 2002).

Chronic Obstructive Pulmonary Disease (COPD). Exposure to respirable silica has also been associated with COPD. COPD is a typically irreversible airflow limita-

---

[5] For examples, see studies on South African gold miners (Hnizdo and Sluis-Cremer, 1993), workers in a U.S. diatomaceous-earth mining and processing facility (Hughes et al., 1998), U.S. hard-rock miners (Kreiss and Zhen, 1996), Canadian gold and uranium miners (Muir et al., 1989a, 1989b), Hong Kong granite workers (Ng and Chan, 1994), U.S. gray-iron foundry workers (Rosenman, Reilly, et al., 1996), and U.S. gold miners (Steenland and Brown, 1995).

[6] Pulmonary tuberculosis is a severe mycobacterial infection caused by the infectious organism *Mycobacterium tuberculosis*. A much higher rate of pulmonary TB among workers with silicosis has been observed in studies on Danish foundry workers (Sherson and Lander, 1990), South African gold miners (Hnizdo and Murray, 1998), California silicosis claimants (Goldsmith et al., 1995), and South African mine workers (Kleinschmidt and Churchyard, 1997).

[7] The least confounded of these studies are based on the following groups of workers: South Dakota gold miners, Danish stone-industry workers, Vermont granite shed and quarry workers, U.S. crushed-stone industry workers, U.S. diatomaceous-earth industry workers, Chinese refractory brick workers, Italian refractory brick workers, UK pottery workers, Chinese pottery workers, and registries of silicotics from North Carolina and Finland (Wilbourn et al., 1997).

tion that frequently results in symptoms that include shortness of breath, coughing, wheezing, and recurrent respiratory infections. Patients diagnosed with COPD usually exhibit some combination of chronic bronchitis, emphysema, and asthma.[8] In a review limited to 13 well-conducted studies of coal miners and South African gold miners, Oxman et al. (1993) concluded that exposure to dust containing silica can cause COPD and that smokers exposed to silica dust are at an increased risk. COPD has also been associated with exposures to other agents, such as fumes and coal dust (Coggon and Taylor, 1998; Harber et al., 2007).

Autoimmune Diseases. Several autoimmune diseases have been associated with inhalation of silica, including scleroderma, systemic lupus erythematosus (lupus), rheumatoid arthritis, autoimmune hemolytic anemia, dermatomyositis or dermatopolymyositis, and several others (NIOSH, 2002). One theory for the association between autoimmune diseases and silica exposure is that the immune system is activated by fibrogenic proteins and growth factors generated by the macrophages produced to extricate the respirable silica particles. An association between autoimmune disease and chronic renal disease following exposure to silica has been detected, but the causal link is unclear.[9]

Occupational Exposure Limits

Workplace exposure limits for crystalline silica were first set by the Occupational Safety and Health Administration (OSHA) in 1972 and vary by type of silica. OSHA's current permissible exposure limit (PEL) time-weighted average (TWA) (PEL-TWA) for all forms of silica in occupational settings is based on a particle-counting method suggested by the American Conference of Governmental Industrial Hygienists (ACGIH)[10] in the 1970s (Yassin, Yebesi, and Tingle, 2005).[11]

---

[8] Emphysema is caused by destruction of the lung parenchyma and results in abnormal enlargement of the air spaces distal to the terminal bronchiole with destructive changes in the alveolar walls. Asthma is "a condition of the lungs in which there is widespread narrowing of the airways" (Stedman, 1990).

[9] To explain the possible effect of silica on the renal system, a direct toxic effect of silica or an immunologic injury by immune-complex formation has been theorized (NIOSH, 2002).

[10] The ACGIH is a membership organization for "all practitioners in industrial hygiene, occupational health, environmental health, and safety domestically and abroad" (ACGIH, 2007). It is not a government agency. The ACGIH is best known for publishing its *Documentation of the Threshold Limit Values* that contains widely accepted exposure limits for chemical substances and physical agents. First published in 1946, the current 7th edition (ACGIH, 2001) includes 642 substances.

[11] OSHA requires that air concentrations of quartz in occupational settings not exceed a TWA concentration of either (250 million particles per cubic foot, or mppcf, $\div$ [% SiO_2 + 5]) or (10 mg/m^3 $\div$ [% SiO_2 + 2]) (as respirable quartz) or 30 mg/m^3 $\div$ (% SiO_2 + 2) (as total quartz), assuming exposures of eight hours per day for a 40-hour workweek (OSHA PEL-TWA) (OSHA, 1997). The limits for cristobalite and tridymite, two other types of crys-

In 1974, NIOSH recommended that occupational exposure limits for crystalline quartz silica be reduced so the respirable fraction of silica-containing dust should not exceed a TWA concentration of more than 0.05 mg/m^3, assuming exposures of up to a 10-hour workday during a 40-hour workweek (recommended exposure limit, or REL, TWA [REL-TWA]) (NIOSH, 2002). At that time, OSHA did not adopt these limits. The exposure limits for silica were revisited in 1988, during the OSHA rulemaking activity on air contaminants, and NIOSH made the same recommendation (NIOSH, 2002). Again, OSHA decided not to adopt the lower limits. In 1986, ACGIH set a TWA concentration limit of 0.10 mg/m^3, assuming exposures of eight hours per day for a 40-hour workweek (ACGIH threshold limit value, time weighted average, or TLV-TWA). Currently, the ACGIH TLV-TWA for respirable crystalline quartz silica is 0.05 mg/m^3 (ACGIH, 2002). However, the ACGIH limits do not have the force of law. OSHA is also currently developing a proposed standard for crystalline silica (OSHA, 2009).

Number of Workers Exposed to Silica

Several attempts have been made to estimate the number of workers in the United States who have been exposed to high levels of silica. Such estimates require historical information on industries with potential silica exposure, including the number of workers and actual measurements of personal exposure to airborne crystalline silica. The most recent of these efforts, conducted by an analyst at OSHA, estimated that a total of 120,000 U.S. workers were "potentially exposed" to crystalline silica, simply based on the number of workers employed in selected industries with a higher risk of exposure to airborne silica over the 16-year period from 1988 to 2003 (Yassin, Yebesi, and Tingle, 2005).[12] However, not all of these workers would be "overexposed" to airborne silica (i.e., exposed to levels above established exposure limits). Based on an analysis of silica exposure measurements from OSHA inspections between 1988 and 2003, Yassin, Yebesi, and Tingle (2005) estimated that 85.5 percent of sampled work-

---

talline silica, are half of those for quartz. In these formulae, %SiO_2 refers to the percentage of crystalline silica (SiO_2), as determined from airborne samples of dust (OSHA, 1997).

[12] Yassin, Yebesi, and Tingle (2005) estimated the number of exposed workers in 18 industries, based on the percentage of their workers exposed to silica, as determined by the OSHA inspector (<1 percent to 30 percent). However, they do not describe the methods used by the OSHA inspector to determine the percentage of workers who were "exposed." The 18 industries included in the analyses were the following standard industrial classification (SIC) codes: metal valves and pipe fittings (3494); special industry machinery (3559); automotive repair paint shop (7532); soap and other detergents (2841); testing laboratory services (8734); gray-iron foundries (3321); manufacturing explosives (2891); fabricated rubber products (3069); masonry and stonework (1741); brick, stone, and related material (5032); repair shops (7699); transmission equipment (3568); chemical preparation (2899); mining machinery equipment (3532); plastic plumbing fixtures (3088); plastering drywall work (1742); tile, marble, and mosaic work (1743); and surgical appliance supplies (3842).

ers were exposed to levels of airborne silica above the ACGIH TLV of 0.05 mg/m^3. However, these study results might not be generalizable because the data analyzed are not a random sample of exposure levels. In addition, the sampling data might overestimate silica exposure because they do not account for use of respirators, and actual exposures might be lower than the ambient readings. Exposure to silica might still continue to occur because almost any process that involves movement of the earth or other disturbances of building products (e.g., bricks, concrete, cement) could expose workers to silica.

Number of Deaths Due to Silicosis

Estimating the numbers of silica-related deaths and diseases is complicated by the long latency periods associated with silica injuries. Typically, 20 to 40 years elapse between the first exposure to silica and disease manifestation (NIOSH, 2002). A study of South African gold miners found, for example, that the average time of first exposure to silica among silicotic miners was 36 years before their diagnosis (Hnizdo and Sluis-Cremer, 1993).

That said, the official count of silicosis-related deaths in the United States stands at 7,642 for the past 35 years combined (from 1968 to 2003).[13] Over that period, the annual count has dropped sixfold; from 1,065 silicosis-related deaths in 1968 to 179 silicosis-related deaths in 2003 (Figure A.1). Throughout the period, about half of these registered deaths had silicosis[14] coded as the underlying (i.e., main) cause of death, while silicosis was a contributing cause on the remainder.[15] To put these numbers in perspective, there were 1,473 deaths in the United States with asbestosis coded as the cause in 2002 (NIOSH, 2005) and 160,440 deaths due to lung cancer in the United States in 2004 (Jemal et al., 2004).

---

[13] The number of silicosis-related deaths occurring in the United States each year from 1968 to 2003 is available from an online query system (National Occupational Respiratory Mortality System, or NORMS) created by NIOSH in 2006. This count is based on the number of death certificates entered in the U.S. vital-statistics registration system with silicosis mentioned as a cause of death. This system generates an official count of deaths based on death certificates from the national vital-statistics registration system. There is a lag period of about three years for summary data on the death statistics (e.g., the count of deaths for 2003 is available in 2006). When the official death statistics are tabulated in NORMS, death certificates with silicosis coded as the underlying cause of death are counted and reported separately from those with silicosis coded as a contributing cause of death.

[14] The code for silicosis is 502 ("Pneumoconiosis due to other silica or silicates") of the International Classification of Diseases, 9th revision, Clinical Modification (ICD-9-CM).

[15] There are two spaces on the death certificate in which the attending physician can record cause-of-death information: the underlying cause of death and the contributing cause(s) of death. If a person has been diagnosed as having silicosis and the physician considers silicosis to be the main reason for the death, silicosis would be recorded as the *underlying* cause of death. If the physician does not consider silicosis to be the main cause of death but thinks it should be mentioned on the death certificate as a factor that contributed to the death, silicosis would be recorded as a *contributing* cause of death.

Figure A.1
Number of Deaths with Any Mention of Silicosis on Death Certificate in the United States, by Year, 1968–2003

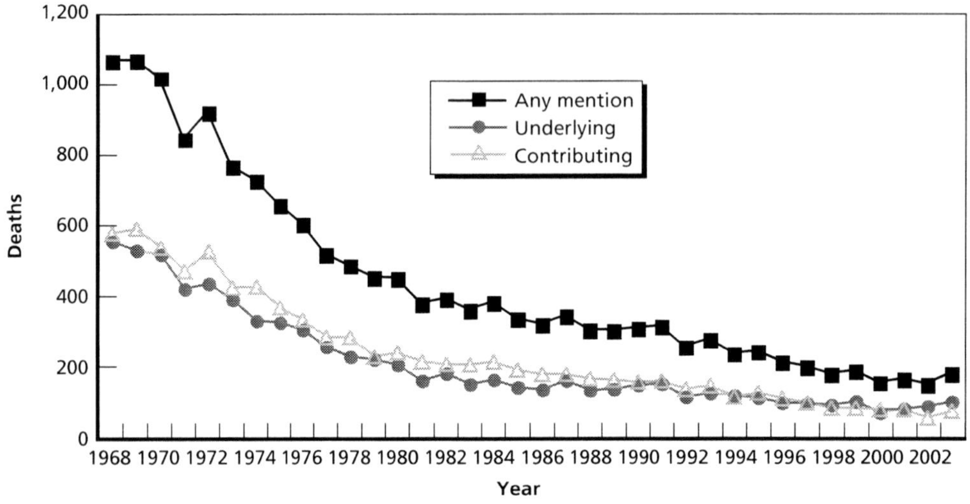

SOURCE: NORMS.
RAND *TR774-A.1*

Deaths attributable at least in part to silicosis are also reported by state. Between 1995 and 2004, silicosis-related deaths were generally stable or decreasing in all states.[16] States with more than ten cases in at least one year during this period include California, Colorado, Michigan, New York, North Carolina, Ohio, Pennsylvania, Texas, and Wisconsin. Pennsylvania and Ohio have the largest number of cases, even though they are not the states with the largest populations. As discussed in Chapter One, a large number of silicosis cases were filed in Mississippi in the early 2000s. The large number of claims stands in contrast to the small number of deaths attributed to silicosis in Mississippi between 1995 and 2004—the number of deaths never exceeded three per year.

Number of Silicosis Cases

There is no accurate measure of how many current and former workers have silicosis.[17] There is also no accurate source of information on how many silicosis cases are

---

[16] Data on state of residence are based on deaths between 1995 and 2004 with silicosis coded as the underlying or contributing cause of death among U.S. residents aged 15 and older (NORMS).

[17] The number of silicosis-related deaths is not a good indicator of the number of people with silicosis because not all people with silicosis die from the disease and because the physician coding the death certificate may not

diagnosed each year in the United States. A surveillance system for tracking occupational illness and injury is operated by the Bureau of Labor Statistics (BLS) of the U.S. Department of Labor. However, this system, which relies on reports from employers, has been found to underestimate the frequency of work-related injuries by 60 percent and work-related illnesses by 66 percent (Rosenman, Kalush, et al., 2006). NIOSH has funded several states to collect data on silicosis cases in one or more years since 1988.[18] Although the NIOSH programs have provided some information each year about new cases of silicosis, there are still no national data collected on the annual number of newly diagnosed silicosis cases and their characteristics.

To address this lack of national data, we applied a method developed by Rosenman, Reilly, and Henneberger (2003) to estimate the number of new silicosis cases occurring in the United States by year. Rosenman's method utilizes data from death certificates and the Michigan silicosis surveillance system, together with a statistical method known as *capture-recapture* to estimate newly diagnosed cases of silicosis in the United States. The method applies several adjustment factors in its calculations. The first step of the calculations excludes the proportion of the silicosis-related deaths that are not confirmed as being silicosis-related (0.2273) according to data from the Michigan silicosis surveillance program. The second step inflates the number of silicosis-related deaths severalfold to account for the fact that not all silicotics die from silicosis. The third step is aimed at inflating the number to account for the fact that surveillance programs are not able to identify all cases of silicosis. The fourth and final step adds the number of silicosis-related deaths and the number of silicosis cases, both calculated by this method, to estimate the total number of newly recognized cases for a given year. By using a range of values as input for these estimates, the method calculates upper and lower bounds for the annual number of silicosis cases for the entire United States.

Based on the fact that 1,065 silicosis-related deaths occurred in the United States during 1968, Rosenman's method projects that between 14,000 and 28,000 new silicosis cases were diagnosed in the United States in that one year alone. As the number of silicosis-related deaths drops from 1968 to 2003, so does the estimated number of new silicosis cases (see Figure A.2). For 2003, the most recent year with available data on silicosis-related deaths, Rosenman's method projects that there were somewhere between 2,400 and 4,700 newly recognized silicosis cases. For comparison, recall that there were 179 deaths with silicosis listed as the underlying or contributing cause in the United States in 2003. The estimates of newly recognized cases should be used with

---

know that the decedent had silicosis. Silicosis researcher Kenneth Rosenman believes that silicosis-related deaths account for about 4 to 8 percent of the silicosis cases each year (Nash, 2004).

[18] Data collection has been funded by NIOSH through its Sentinel Event Notification System for Occupational Risks (SENSOR) program in California, Illinois, Michigan, New Jersey, New Mexico, New York, North Carolina, Ohio, Texas, and Wisconsin. However, Michigan and New Jersey were the only states funded in 2007 (NIOSH, 2008).

Figure A.2
Estimated Number of New Silicosis Cases in the United States, by Year, 1968–2003

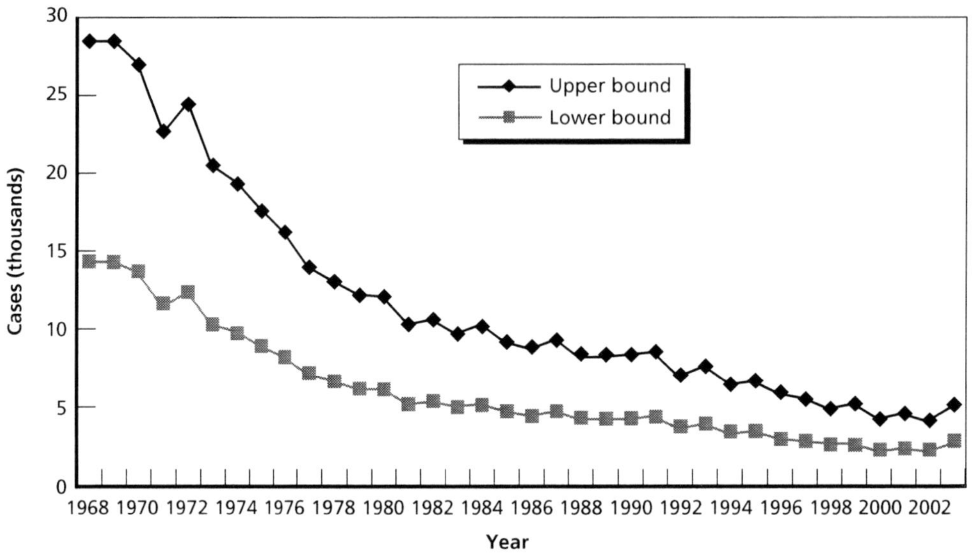

SOURCE: NORMS.

RAND *TR774-A.2*

caution, given that they are based on several assumptions that might not all hold or that might change over time.

Several issues should be kept in mind when projecting the occurrence of silicosis into the future. First, as mentioned earlier, silicosis can be diagnosed long after a person is exposed to silica (NIOSH, 2002). Second, silicosis can occur following exposure to levels at or under the OSHA PEL (NIOSH, 2002). Third, concentrations of respirable crystalline silica might be higher than industrial hygiene measurements indicate because it is technically difficult to measure (NIOSH, 2002). In addition, occupational exposure to silica is not easily controlled because some industries in which silica is found (e.g., construction) are not easily subjected to engineering controls (NIOSH, 2002). Because of all of these factors, many occupational exposures might exceed federal standards (NIOSH, 2002), resulting in the occurrence of silicosis many years into the future.

Conclusion

A review of the available scientific literature suggests that death and disease due to silica exposure in the workplace have declined substantially in the past 40 years. However, it appears that silica exposure remains an ongoing threat to health in the workplace. Thousands of workers may still be exposed to silica levels that exceed NIOSH's REL each year. The estimated number of new silicosis cases dropped substantially between 1968 and 2003, but we project that there may still be on the order of 2,000 to 5,000 new silicosis cases diagnosed per year in the United States. Deaths due at least in part to silica also dropped substantially in the same period, but close to 200 silicosis-related deaths continue to be reported each year. These deaths and diagnoses will provide the basis for new silica lawsuits in the coming years.

APPENDIX B

Evolution of Silica Litigation Prior to MDL 1553

As illustrated in Appendix A, medical practitioners and health researchers have long been aware of the dangers of silica dust. Likewise, litigation over compensation for silica-related injuries stretches back to at least to the 1930s. In this appendix, we provide an overview of the litigation between the 1930s and the 1990s.

Silica litigation flared up in the 1930s but was quickly extinguished by the inclusion of silica-related injuries in the workers' compensation programs. Changes in liability doctrine and a number of other factors led to a reemergence of silica litigation in the 1970s, and the number of cases increased gradually though the 1990s.

Appearance of Silica Litigation in the 1930s

During the Great Depression, contemporary observers cited an epidemic of lawsuits that threatened the foundry, mining, quarry, and construction sectors ("Silicosis Menace," 1933). Insurance companies were particularly anxious, seeing the rapid rise in silicosis lawsuits as a risk to the whole industry. Some insurers forced companies to medically screen employees for silicosis and to fire anyone with signs of silicosis, in an effort to contain the crisis. This had little immediate impact, as scores of lawsuits went forward. As Rosner and Markowitz (1991, p. 80) write,

> Faced by conflicting medical testimony about the nature and causes of the plaintiff's lung condition, and faced with the workers' often obvious suffering, jurors in the early years of the Depression frequently brought judgments against insurance companies and industry alike.

As plaintiffs were increasingly successful in court, more workers inflicted with silicosis came forward with suits. In 1933, in New York state alone, more than $30 million worth of lawsuits were filed against industry ("Silicosis Menace," 1933). While it is difficult to measure the magnitude of claims with precision, a contemporary observer noted that the amount typically claimed for an individual rose from $5,000–$10,000 to $100,000 (Tillson, 1934, pp. 19–20).

As silica litigation expanded, issues about diagnoses arose. While the early suits were brought largely by sick workers, the successive waves of lawsuits were also made up of litigants who were not currently sick but who had x-ray evidence (or, in some cases, diagnoses) showing that they had early-stage silicosis: a physical change to the lungs but often without any present impairment in ability to work. Many of these cases resulted in verdicts favoring the plaintiffs.

The Hawk's Nest tunnel disaster was perhaps the zenith of silica litigation in the 1930s. The incident involved construction of a dam and large tunnel near a mountain called Hawk's Nest in West Virginia. The tunnel was designed to feed a hydropower plant and was drilled through almost pure silica. Workers were exposed to extreme concentrations of silica, and many filed suit once reports of an unusual number of deaths began emerging. The first Hawk's Nest suits were filed in 1932, and, ultimately, 336 suits were brought against the primary contractor for the project. The Hawk's Nest incident had ramifications in several dimensions. The threat of ongoing litigation prompted the West Virginia House of Delegates to add silicosis to the list of conditions covered by the workers' compensation system in 1935. Newspaper and press attention raised awareness of the dangers of silica, as did congressional hearings in 1936 on the risks associated with silica exposure.[1]

The Shift into Workers' Compensation

Most states adopted workers' compensation systems for most industrial accidents between 1910 and 1920 (Fishback and Kantor, 2000). While not uniformly popular with employers,[2] they had the virtue of replacing an often inconsistent system of tort law with a system that more reliably provided compensation for the many injured in industrial accidents. The exclusive-remedy provisions of most workers' compensation laws also shielded the employer from suit.

It was not clear to many commentators at the time whether the workers' compensation system was an appropriate outlet for compensation for long-latency diseases like silicosis—workers' compensation had been initially established with the expectation that it would cover industrial accidents. Long-latency diseases were often difficult to tie to a particular cause, and a mobile workforce meant that tying a disease to a particular employer was also difficult. For these reasons, silicosis and many other diseases were not initially covered by workers' compensation.

[1] For detailed accounts of the Hawk's Nest incident and its aftermath, see Cherniack (1986) and Rosner and Markowitz (1991).

[2] Workers' compensation programs were initially quite controversial and, at times, industrial defendants successfully challenged them on constitutional grounds. See, e.g. *Ives v. South B. R. Co.* (1911).

With the rise of the silica litigation, however, employers and insurers began to view workers' compensation as an attractive means to reduce liability. In 1934, efforts to push silicosis into the workers' compensation system began in earnest in New York. As New York industrial commissioner Elmer Andrews (1936) stated later,

> employers who had opposed the inclusion of silicosis under the Workmen's Compensation Law, came running to the state pleading for the inclusion of silicosis under the Workmen's Compensation Act so that they would be protected against the unlimited and terrifying common law damage suits which were being filed against them.

By late in the year, the New York statute had been amended to include all industrial diseases, which prevented workers from directly bringing silica suits against their employers.

The experience with the earlier increase in tort cases by plaintiffs who had been diagnosed with silicosis but were not currently sick led industry and insurance leaders to seek a requirement that a worker must show that his or her ability to work was impaired in order to receive workers' compensation benefits. The debate over whether unimpaired workers (workers who had silicosis but could still work) should be compensated was hotly debated. Labor argued that the approach of defining compensable silicosis as requiring disability ignored those who would become disabled upon retirement. Businesses, in contrast, feared that the workers' compensation system would be turned into universal health insurance. Eventually, New York policymakers decided that a laborer must be suffering from medically diagnosed silicosis-related shortness of breath to qualify for workers' compensation.[3] Silicosis alone, without an accompanying decreased capacity to work, would not constitute a disability for purposes of the workers' compensation statutes (Rosner and Markowitz, 1991, p. 90).

Expanding workers' compensation to include industrial disease had the effect of dramatically increasing workers' compensation insurance rates. Some insurers announced that they were raising rates by as much as 400 percent and required employers to screen employees for silicosis and to fire silicotic workers before the expansion of workers' compensation went into effect. As a result of these developments, new legislation was passed in New York that greatly restricted compensation. No compensation was provided for partial disability, and compensation for total disability could not exceed $3,000 (Rosner and Markowitz, 1991, p. 93). In the environment of the Great Depression, many labor unions chose to support this legislation, fearing that opposi-

[3] Parallels to recent controversies about who should be entitled to recover for silicosis (and asbestos) are striking. See Carroll et al. (2005), discussing recovery for unimpaired asbestotics.

tion might cost members their jobs. By the end of 1939, only 79 workers filed silicosis workers' compensation claims in New York and received a total of less than $100,000.[4]

After World War II, there was little litigation over injuries due to silica dust. Social security and unemployment insurance provided a safety net that an earlier generation of silicotic workers lacked. Union-management agreements in the postwar era led to widespread provision of health insurance for unionized workers. As a result of new antibiotics, mortality risk from TB exacerbated by silicosis declined (Rosner and Markowitz, 1991, p. 221), though congressional hearings in the mid-1950s still indicated disproportionately high TB in mining areas with high numbers of silicotics (U.S. Congress, 1956, p. 409).[5] Perhaps most importantly, the exclusive-remedy provisions and inclusion of silicosis as a compensable condition in workers' compensation laws eliminated the primary defendants from liability. At the same time, engineering controls in workplaces became more common and gradually improved.

The Reemergence of Silica Litigation in the 1970s

After decades of quiet, silica litigation began to reemerge in the 1970s. Figure B.1 shows the growth in claims filed against U.S. Silica, a major national silica manufacturer. Small numbers of tort cases began to appear in the 1970s, increasing gradually to roughly 50 per year in the second half of the 1980s and first half of the 1990s (except for a spike in Cambria County, Pennsylvania, in 1987).[6] Claims jumped to much higher levels in second half of the 1990s, averaging about 530 claims per year between 1995 and 1999.

Figure B.1 shows the high proportion of claims against this manufacturer that were filed in Texas. Between 1975 and 1999, 62 percent of the 2,969 claims filed against U.S. Silica were filed in Texas, far exceeding the proportion of the firm's sand deliveries in Texas in the latter part of this period.[7] While data from other manufacturers are needed to determine whether silica litigation from 1985 through 1999 was, in large part, a Texas phenomenon, Texas was clearly an important venue for litigation. Presaging the events to come, Figure B.1 also shows a spike in claims in Mississippi

[4] According to Rosner and Markowitz (1991), the history of silica litigation and legislation shifting silicosis into workers' compensation was similar in other states.

[5] See also discussion of silicosis mortality rates in Chapter Two.

[6] Missing from the U.S. Silica data are claims related to litigation involving the Lynchburg Foundry (in Virginia) in the early 1980s.

[7] Deliveries in Texas accounted for about 14 percent of total shipments nationwide between 1992 and 1999 (U.S. Silica, 2006). Most relevant to silica claims in the late 1990s would be exposures and sand deliveries in earlier years due to the long latency periods associated with silicosis. However, data are not available by state for earlier shipments.

Figure B.1
Claims Against U.S. Silica, 1975–1999

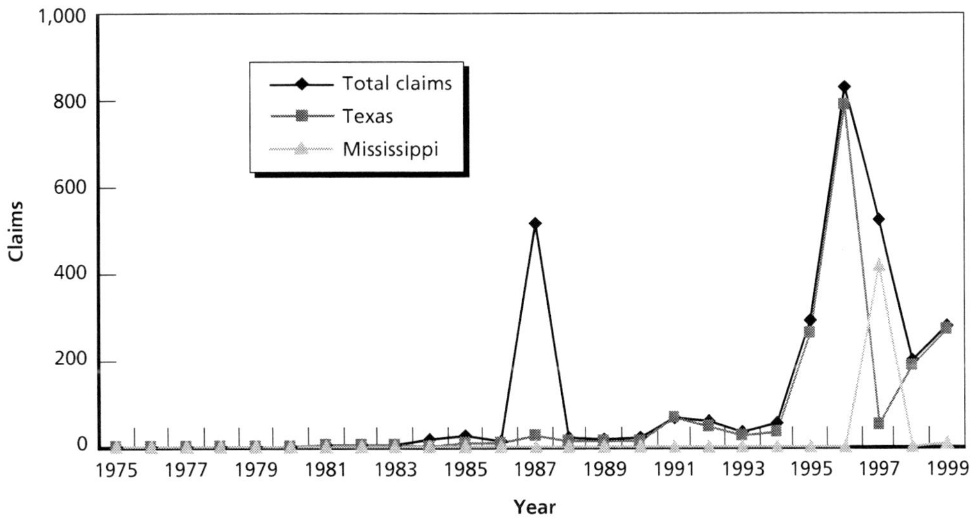

SOURCE: U.S. Silica (2007).
RAND *TR774-B.1*

in 1997. Together, claims filed in Mississippi and Texas account for nearly the entire increase in silica claims filed against U.S. Silica in the second half of the 1990s.

The increase in silica claims between the 1970s and the 1990s was due to a number of different factors, likely including

- increased awareness of the exposure to respirable silica
- changes in legal doctrine
- limited compensation under workers' compensation
- asbestos litigation.

We discuss each factor in turn.

Increased Awareness of the Incidence of Silicosis

Soon after its creation in 1970, NIOSH undertook a study to examine silicosis—thought to be easy because it was a "disease of the past." However, the study discovered that silicosis was still a major threat to industrial workers (NIOSH, 1974). This led to the agency's unsuccessful attempt to revise the acceptable threshold for silica exposure among industrial workers (see Appendix A). NIOSH also suggested banning silica sand for use in abrasive blasting altogether as had long been the case in Europe. In 1977, OSHA attempted to totally ban silica sand for use in abrasive blasting. The sandblasting and sand-producer industries fought this effort and argued that the data were not clear and that adequate safety equipment could minimize the risk from silica. After several delays in the late 1970s, the Ronald Reagan administration ultimately abandoned the attempt to impose new standards.

Other public-health research also contributed to increased awareness of silica as a public-health threat. In 1997, the IARC classified silica as a group 1 carcinogen. In addition, there was growing evidence that exposure was tied to several autoimmune diseases, including rheumatoid arthritis, lupus, scleroderma, and renal disease (Steenland and Goldsmith, 1995).

The creation of OSHA and NIOSH and related public-health research created an increased awareness of occupational-safety issues in general and the risk of silica in particular. This increased awareness may have been one factor behind the increase in silica litigation.

Changes in Legal Doctrine

Expansions in legal doctrine that began in the 1960s made it possible for workers to sue silica and protective-equipment manufacturers, rather than their employers, for workplace injuries. A precedent-setting federal appeals court decision in 1973 opened the way for asbestos workers to sue product manufacturers based on failing to warn either the employer or the employee of the dangers of asbestos (*Borel v. Fibreboard Paper Products Corp.*, 1974). The decision was applied in silica and other settings with the consequence that the exclusive-remedy provisions of the workers' compensation system still largely prevented silica suits against the employer but no longer wholly prevented silica lawsuits.

Limited Compensation Under Workers' Compensation

Dissatisfaction by workers and their advocates with both the amount of benefits available through the workers' compensation system and the difficulties of accessing those benefits may have also contributed to the reemergence of silica litigation. Workers' compensation provides only partial compensation for workplace injuries. Unlike the tort system, under workers' compensation, pain and suffering are not compensable. In addition, workers' compensation programs do not fully replace wage loss, in part because workers' compensation benefits are not taxable and in part to retain incentives to return to work (see Biddle, Boden, and Reville, 2001, p. 276).

The long latency period of most silica injuries likely increased the difficulty of accessing workers' compensation benefits. The availability of benefits is straightforward for traumatic injuries that occur in the workplace. In contrast, it may be difficult to establish eligibility for benefits when a worker with newly diagnosed silicosis has long been retired or no longer works where the silica exposure took place. The complexities of accessing workers' compensation for a latent injury related to silica exposure may thus have the net effect of reducing or eliminating the compensation available from the workers' compensation system.

Losses that remain uncompensated, either due to difficulties accessing the program or the compensation schedule, provide a powerful incentive to turn to the tort system for compensation.

Asbestos Litigation

Application of the expanded liability in the industrial-dust context was pioneered through asbestos litigation. The success of asbestos litigation against third-party defendants provided a legal and business model that plaintiffs' firms specializing in silica litigation could follow (see generally Carroll et al., 2005). The expertise, strategies, financial resources, and connections with medical screening firms and diagnosis-providing doctors accumulated by plaintiffs' attorneys during asbestos litigation set the stage for the rise in silica litigation. Indeed, many of the leading lawyers, medical screening firms, and diagnosis-providing doctors in silica litigation had previously been very active in asbestos litigation.

Conclusion

Compensation for silica injuries has bounced between the tort system and the workers' compensation system. Silica-related injuries were initially thought inappropriate for inclusion in early workers' compensation programs. A spurt of litigation in the 1930s then led policymakers to conclude that workers' compensation was, after all, preferable to tort for silica injuries. Tort litigation over silica-related injuries consequently disappeared for more than three decades. The increased awareness of silica exposure as a ongoing public-health problem, the less-than-full compensation provided by workers' compensation, changes in legal doctrine that allowed third-party claims for workplace injuries under certain circumstances, and the practices and relationships developed in asbestos litigation all likely contributed in varying degrees to the reemergence of silica tort litigation in the 1970s.

References

ACGIH—*see* American Conference of Governmental Industrial Hygienists.

Acuna v. Brown and Root Inc., 200 F.3d 335, 5th Cir., January 11, 2000.

Alexander v. Air Liquide America Corp., No. 03-533, S.D. Tex., 2005.

American Conference of Governmental Industrial Hygienists, *Documentation of the Threshold Limit Values and Biological Exposure Indices*, 7th ed., Cincinnati, Ohio, 2001.

———, *Guide to Occupational Exposure Values, 2002*, Cincinnati, Ohio, 2002.

———, "About: History," last updated May 15, 2007. As of September 13, 2006: http://www.acgih.org/about/history.htm

American Thoracic Society, "Adverse Effects of Crystalline Silica Exposure," *American Journal of Respiratory and Critical Care Medicine*, Vol. 155, 1997, pp. 761–765. As of October 17, 2009: http://www.thoracic.org/sections/publications/statements/pages/eoh/506.html

Andrews, Elmer, industrial commissioner, testimony before New York State Senate Labor and Industries Committee, National Archives, Record Group 100, 7-2-1-5-1, March 31, 1936.

Austern, David, president, Claims Resolution Management Corporation, "Suspension of Acceptance of Medical Records," memorandum, September 12, 2005.

Behrens, Mark A., and Phil Goldberg, "The Asbestos Litigation Crisis: The Tide Appears to Be Turning," *Connecticut Insurance Law Journal,* Vol. 12, No. 2, 2005–2006.

Behrens, Mark A., Leah Lorber, and Cary Silverman, "Silica: An Overview of Exposure and Litigation in the United States," *LexisNexis Mealey's Litigation Report: Asbestos*, Vol. 20, No. 2, February 21, 2005.

Biddle, Jeff E., Leslie I. Boden, and Robert T. Reville, "Permanent Partial Disability from Occupational Injuries: Earnings Losses and Replacement in Three States," in Peter P. Budetti, Richard V. Burkhauser, Janice M. Gregory, and H. Allan Hunt, eds., *Ensuring Health and Income Security for an Aging Workforce*, Kalamazoo, Mich.: W. E. Upjohn Institute for Employment Research, 2001, pp. 263–290.

Borel v. Fibreboard Paper Products Corp., 493 F.2d 1076, 5th Cir., May 13, 1974.

Carroll, Stephen J., Deborah Hensler, Jennifer Gross, Elizabeth M. Sloss, Matthias Schonlau, Allan Abrahamse, and J. Scott Ashwood, *Asbestos Litigation*, Santa Monica, Calif.: RAND Corporation, MG-162-ICJ, 2005. As of October 16, 2009: http://www.rand.org/pubs/monographs/MG162/

Cherniack, Martin, *The Hawk's Nest Incident: America's Worst Industrial Disaster*, New Haven, Conn.: Yale University Press, 1986.

Coggon, David, and Anthony Newman Taylor, "Coal Mining and Chronic Obstructive Pulmonary Disease: A Review of the Evidence," *Thorax*, Vol. 53, 1998, pp. 398–407.

Constitution of the Commonwealth of Massachusetts, June 15, 1780. As of October 17, 2009: http://www.mass.gov/legis/const.htm

Daniels, Stephen, and Joanne Martin, "Texas Plaintiffs' Practice in the Age of Tort Reform: Survival of the Fittest—It's Even More True Now," *New York Law School Law Review*, Vol. 51, 2006–2007.

Daubert v. Merrell Dow Pharms., 509 U.S. 579, 113 S. Ct. 2786, June 28, 1993.

Davies, Paul, "Class Inaction: Plaintiffs' Lawsuits Against Companies Sharply Declines," *Wall Street Journal*, August 26, 2006, p. A1.

Dixon, Lloyd, and Brian Gill, *Changes in the Standards for Admitting Expert Evidence in Federal Civil Cases Since the Daubert Decision*, Santa Monica, Calif.: RAND Corporation, MR-1439-ICJ, 2001. As of November 10, 2009:
http://www.rand.org/pubs/monograph_reports/MR1439/

Dublin, Louis I., "Conditions of Industry Which Unfavorably Affect the Health of Workers," *Eighth Annual New York State Industrial Conference Proceedings*, Albany, N.Y.: J. B. Lyon, Co., 1925.

Dubos, René J., and Jean Dubos, *The White Plague: Tuberculosis, Man, and Society*, New Brunswick, N.J.: Rutgers University Press, 1952 (1987).

Federal Judicial Center, *Manual for Complex Litigation, Fourth*, St. Paul, Minn., 2004.

Federal Rules of Civil Procedure, Rule 11, Signing Pleadings, Motions, and Other Papers; Representations to the Court; Sanctions.

———, Rule 42, Consolidation; Separate Trials.

Fishback, Price Van Meter, and Shawn Everett Kantor, *A Prelude to the Welfare State: The Origins of Workers' Compensation*, Chicago, Ill.: University of Chicago Press, 2000.

Frye v. United States, 293 F. 1013, 54 App. D.C. 46, December 3, 1923.

Gibbes, Heneage, "Is the Unity of Phthisis an Established Fact? An Important Consideration in Regard to the Cure of the Disease by Inoculation," *Boston Medical and Surgical Journal*, December 25, 1890, Vol. 123, p. 608.

Glater, Jonathan D., "Asbestos Fund Bars 9 Doctors," *New York Times*, September 15, 2005. As of October 16, 2009:
http://www.nytimes.com/2005/09/15/business/15asbestos.html

Goldsmith, David F., James J. Beaumont, Lynne A. Morrin, and Marc B. Schenker, "Respiratory Cancer and Other Chronic Disease Mortality Among Silicotics in California," *American Journal of Industrial Medicine*, Vol. 28, No. 4, October 1995, pp. 459–467.

Harber, Philip, Donald P. Tashkin, Michael Simmons, Lori Crawford, Eva Hnizdo, and John Connett, "Effect of Occupational Exposures on Decline of Lung Function in Early Chronic Obstructive Pulmonary Disease," *American Journal of Respiratory and Critical Care Medicine*, Vol. 176, 2007, pp. 994–1000.

Hayhurst, Emery Roe, *Consumption and Preventable Deaths in American Occupations*, Columbus, Ohio: Heer Printing Co., 1914.

Hnizdo, Eva, and J. Murray, "Risk of Pulmonary Tuberculosis Relative to Silicosis and Exposure to Silica Dust in South African Gold Miners," *Occupational and Environmental Medicine*, Vol. 55, No. 7, July 1998, pp. 496–502.

Hnizdo, Eva, and G. K. Sluis-Cremer, "Risk of Silicosis in a Cohort of White South African Gold Miners," *American Journal of Industrial Medicine*, Vo. 24, No. 4, October 1993, pp. 447–457.

Hoffman, Frederick L., and S. E. Forman, "Mortality from Consumption in Dusty Trades: Charity Relief and Wage Earnings," *Bulletin of the Bureau of Labor*, No. 79, November 1908, pp. 633–875.

Hughes, Janet M., Hans Weill, Harvey Checkoway, Robert N. Jones, Melanie M. Henry, Nicholas J. Heyer, Noah S. Seixas, and Paul A. Demers, "Radiographic Evidence of Silicosis Risk in the Diatomaceous Earth Industry," *American Journal of Respiratory and Critical Care Medicine*, Vol. 158, No. 3, September 1998, pp. 807–814.

IARC—*see* International Agency for Research on Cancer.

ICM-9-CM—*see* U.S. Health Care Financing Administration, National Center for Health Statistics, Centers for Medicare and Medicaid Services, and Centers for Disease Control and Prevention.

In re Silica Products Liability Litigation, 398 F. Supp. 2d 563, S.D. Tex., MDL 1553, September 30, 2005. As of October 16, 2009:
http://www.txs.uscourts.gov/notablecases/203md1553/

International Agency for Research on Cancer, Working Group on the Evaluation of Carcinogenic Risks to Humans, *Silica, Some Silicates, Coal Dust, and Para-Aramid Fibrils*, Vol. 68, Lyon, France, 1997.

Ives v. South B. R. Co., 201 N.Y. 271, 94 N.E. 431, Ct. App. N.Y., March 24, 1911.

Jemal, Ahmedin, Ram C. Tiwari, Taylor Murray, Asma Ghafoor, Alicia Samuels, Elizabeth Ward, Eric J. Feuer, and Michael J. Thun, "Cancer Statistics 2004," *CA Cancer Journal for Clinicians*, Vol. 54, No. 1, January–February 2004, pp. 8–29.

Kleinschmidt, I., and G. Churchyard, "Variation in Incidences of Tuberculosis in Subgroups of South African Gold Miners," *Occupational and Environmental Medicine*, Vol. 54, No. 9, September 1997, pp. 636–641.

Kreiss, Kathleen, and Boguang Zhen, "Risk of Silicosis in a Colorado Mining Community," *American Journal of Industrial Medicine*, Vol. 30, No. 5, November 1996, pp. 529–539.

"Law Firms Won't Be Sanctioned Over Silica Screenings," *Andrews Toxic Tort Litigation Reporter*, November 2007.

Lore v. Lone Pine Corp., 1986 N.J. Super. LEXIS 1626, November 18, 1986.

Manville Trust, claim history provided to the authors by Claims Resolution Management Co., August 2007.

Massachusetts Constitution—*see* Constitution of the Commonwealth of Massachusetts.

MDL 1553—*see In re Silica Products Liability Litigation.*

Muir, D. C. F., H. S. Shannon, J. A. Julian, D. K. Verma, A. Sebestyen, and Charles D. Bernholz, "Silica Exposure and Silicosis Among Ontario Hardrock Miners, I. Methodology," *American Journal of Industrial Medicine*, Vol. 16, No. 1, 1989a, pp. 5–11.

———, "Silica Exposure and Silicosis Among Ontario Hardrock Miners, III: Analysis and Risk Estimates," *American Journal of Industrial Medicine*, Vol. 16, 1989b, pp. 29–43.

Nash, James, "Why Are So Many Workers Still Exposed to Silica?" *EHS Today*, November 16, 2004. As of October 18, 2009:
http://ehstoday.com/ppe/respirators/ehs_imp_37292/

National Institute for Occupational Safety and Health, *Occupational Exposure to Crystalline Silica: Criteria for a Recommended Standard*, Washington, D.C., NIOSH 75-120, 1974. As of October 17, 2009:
http://www.cdc.gov/niosh/pdfs/75-120a.pdf

———, *Request for Assistance in Preventing Silicosis and Deaths from Sandblasting*, Cincinnati, Ohio: U.S. Department of Health and Human Services, Public Health Service, Centers for Disease Control, National Institute for Occupational Safety and Health, NIOSH 92-102, August 1992. As of February 4, 2008:
http://www.cdc.gov/Niosh/92-102.html

———, *Health Effects of Occupational Exposure to Respirable Crystalline Silica*, Cincinnati, Ohio: U.S. Department of Health and Human Services, Centers for Disease Control and Prevention, National Institute for Occupational Safety and Health, NIOSH 2002-129, 2002. As of November 2, 2009:
http://www.cdc.gov/niosh/docs/2002-129/02-129a.html

———, "Asbestosis: Number of Deaths by Sex, Race, and Age, and Median Age at Death, U.S. Residents Age 15 and Over, 1993–2002," *Work-Related Lung Disease (WoRLD) Surveillance System*, Table 2005T01-01, c. 2005. As of February 5, 2009:
http://www2.cdc.gov/drds/worldreportdata/gif/2005Table01-01.gif

———, "State-Based Surveillance Programs," last reviewed December 5, 2008. As of July 31, 2007:
http://www.cdc.gov/niosh/topics/surveillance/ords/StateBasedSurveillance/Stateprograms.html#states

———, "National Occupational Respiratory Mortality System," last reviewed May 14, 2009. As of July 31, 2007:
http://webappa.cdc.gov/ords/norms.html

Ng, Tze-Pin, and Shiu-Lun Chan, "Quantitative Relations Between Silica Exposure and Development of Radiological Small Opacities in Granite Workers," *Annals of Occupational Hygiene*, Vol. 38, Supp. 1, 1994, pp. 857–863.

Ng, Tze-Pin, Shiu-Lun Chan, and Ka-Ping Lam, "Radiological Progression and Lung Function in Silicosis: A Ten Year Follow Up Study," *British Medical Journal*, Vol. 295, July 18, 1987, pp. 164–168.

NIOSH—*see* National Institute for Occupational Safety and Health.

NORMS—*see* National Institute for Occupational Safety and Health (2009).

Occupational Safety and Health Administration, "Mineral Dusts: 1910.1000 Table Z-3," *General Industry: OSHA Safety and Health Standards (29 CFR 1910)*, Washington, D.C., 1997. As of October 18, 2009:
http://www.osha.gov/pls/oshaweb/owadisp.show_document?p_table=standards&p_id=9994

———, "Occupational Safety and Health Administration Peer Review Agenda," last updated June 15, 2009. As of November 11, 2009:
http://www.osha.gov/dsg/peer_review/peer_agenda.html

Oliver, Thomas, *Dangerous Trades: The Historical, Social, and Legal Aspects of Industrial Occupations as Affecting Health, by a Number of Experts*, London: J. Murray, 1902.

Order No. 29, Addressing Subject-Matter Jurisdiction, Expert Testimony and Sanctions, *In re Silica Products Liability Litigation*, S.D. Tex., June 30, 2005. As of October 16, 2009:
http://www.txs.uscourts.gov/notablecases/203md1553/203md1553-1902.pdf

OSHA—*see* Occupational Safety and Health Administration.

Oxman, A. D., D. C. F. Muir, H. S. Shannon, S. R. Stock, E. Hnizdo, and H. J. Lange, "Occupational Dust Exposure and Chronic Obstructive Pulmonary Disease: A Systematic Overview of the Evidence," *American Review of Respiratory Disease*, Vol. 148, No. 1, July 1993, pp. 38–48.

Ransome, Arthur, *The Causes and Prevention of Phthisis*, London: Smith, Elder, 1890.

Rosenman, Kenneth D., Alice Kalush, Mary Jo Reilly, Joseph C. Gardiner, Mathew Reeves, and Zhewui Luo, "How Much Work-Related Injury and Illness Is Missed by the Current National Surveillance System?" *Journal of Occupational and Environmental Medicine*, Vol. 48, No. 4, April 2006, pp. 357–365.

Rosenman, Kenneth D., E. Pechter, D. P. Schill, D. J. Valiante, E. A. Bresnitz, K. R. Cummings, E. Socie, and M. S. Filios, "Silicosis in Dental Laboratory Technicians: Five States, 1994–2000," *MMWR Weekly*, Vol. 53, No. 9, March 12, 2004, pp. 195–197. As of October 17, 2009: http://www.cdc.gov/mmwr/preview/mmwrhtml/mm5309a3.htm

Rosenman, Kenneth D., Mary Jo Reilly, and Paul K. Henneberger, "Estimating the Total Number of Newly-Recognized Silicosis Cases in the United States," *American Journal of Industrial Medicine*, Vol. 44, No. 2, 2003, pp. 141–147.

Rosenman, Kenneth D., Mary Jo Reilly, Carol Rice, Vicki Hertzberg, Chih-Yu Tseng, and Henry A. Anderson, "Silicosis Among Foundry Workers: Implication for the Need to Revise the OSHA Standard," *American Journal of Epidemiology*, Vol. 144, No. 9, 1996, pp. 890–900.

Rosner, David, and Gerald E. Markowitz, *Deadly Dust: Silicosis and the Politics of Occupational Disease in Twentieth-Century America*, Princeton, N.J.: Princeton University Press, 1991.

Sherson, D., and F. Lander, "Morbidity of Pulmonary Tuberculosis Among Silicotic and Nonsilicotic Foundry Workers in Denmark," *Journal of Occupational Medicine*, Vol. 32, No. 2, February 1990, pp. 110–113.

"Silicosis Menace," *Business Week*, September 1933, pp. 19–20.

Stedman, Thomas Lathrop, *Stedman's Medical Dictionary*, 25th ed., Baltimore, Md.: Williams and Wilkins, 1990.

Steenland, Kyle, and David Brown, "Silicosis Among Gold Miners: Exposure—Response Analyses and Risk Assessment," *American Journal of Public Health*, Vol. 85, No. 10, October 1995, pp. 1372–1377.

Steenland, Kyle, and D. Goldsmith, "Silica Exposure and Autoimmune Diseases," *American Journal of Industrial Medicine*, Vol. 28, No. 5, November 1995, pp. 603–608.

Tillson, Benjamin F., "Silicosis: Its Economic Aspects," *Engineering and Mining Journal*, June 1934.

U.S. Code, Title 28, Judiciary and Judicial Procedure, Part IV, Jurisdiction and Venue, Chapter 87, District Courts: Venue, Section 1407, Multidistrict Litigation.

———, Title 28, Judiciary and Judicial Procedure, Part V, Procedure, Chapter 123, Fees and Costs, Section 1927, Counsel's Liability for Excessive Costs.

U.S. Congress, 84th Cong., 2nd Sess., House Subcommittee on Mine Safety of the Committee on Education and Labor, hearings on inspection and investigation in metallic mines, 1956.

U.S. Health Care Financing Administration, National Center for Health Statistics, Centers for Medicare and Medicaid Services, and Centers for Disease Control and Prevention, *The International Classification of Diseases, Clinical Modification: ICD-CM*, 9th rev., 6th ed., Baltimore, Md., October 2009. As of October 18, 2009:
http://purl.access.gpo.gov/GPO/LPS8749

U.S. Silica, data on tons of silica shipped by state, provided to authors, 2006.

———, data on silica claims from 1975 through June 2007, provided to authors, 2007.

Warner, John Harley, *The Therapeutic Perspective: Medical Practice, Knowledge, and Identity in America, 1820–1885*, Cambridge, Mass.: Harvard University Press, 1986.

White, Michelle J., "Asbestos and the Future of Mass Torts," *Journal of Economic Perspectives*, Vol. 18, No. 2, Spring 2004, pp. 183–204. As of October 16, 2009: http://weber.ucsd.edu/~miwhite/asbestos-jep-final.pdf

Wilbourn, Julian D., Douglas B. McGregor, Christiane Partensky, and Jerry M. Rice, "IARC Reevaluates Silica and Related Substances," *Environmental Health Perspectives*, Vol. 105, No. 7, July 1997, pp. 756–759.

Yablon, Charles, "Hindsight, Regret, and Safe Harbors in Rule 11 Litigation," *Loyola of Los Angeles Law Review*, Vol. 37, No. 3, Winter 2004, pp. 599–644. As of October 23, 2009: http://llr.lls.edu/volumes/v37-issue3/documents/yablon.pdf.pdf

Yassin, Abdiaziz, Francis Yebesi, and Rex Tingle, "Occupational Exposure to Crystalline Silica Dust in the United States, 1988–2003," *Environmental Health Perspectives*, Vol. 113, No. 3, March 2005, pp. 255–260.